GERIATRIC CARE
IN
ADVANCED SOCIETIES

Geriatric Care in Advanced Societies

Edited by

J C Brocklehurst, MD, MSc, FRCP

Professor of Geriatric Medicine, University of Manchester

Published by
MTP
P.O. Box 55,
St. Leonard's House,
St. Leonard's Gate,
Lancaster.

Softcover reprint of the hardcover 1st edition 1975

ISBN-13: 978-94-011-7172-4 e-ISBN-13: 978-94-011-7170-0
DOI: 10.1007/978-94-011-7170-0

Contents

List of contributors

Ms Irene M Burnside
Ethel Percy Andras Gerontology Center
University of Southern California
California, Los Angeles, USA

Professor J C Brocklehurst
Professor of Geriatric Medicine
University of Manchester
England

Dr R M Gibson
Regional Geriatrician,
NSW Health Commission—
Hunter Health Commission
Seconded from Royal Newcastle Hospital
Newcastle, New South Wales
Australia

Dr R G Revutskaya
Chief
Operational Research Department, Institute of Gerontology AMS USSR,
Kiev, USSR

Dr Isadore Rossman
Medical Director
Home Care and
Extended Services Department
Montefiore Hospital, New York
Associate Professor of
Community Medicine
Albert Einstein College of Medicine, Bronx, New York,
USA

Dr Alvar Svanborg
Chairman of Vasa Hospital
Head of Clinic II
University of Goteborg, Sweden

Dr R J van Zonneveld
Director
Bureau Raad voor
Gezondheidsresearch TNO
(Council for Health Research TNO), The Hague

CHAPTER ONE

Introduction: the development of geriatric care in advanced societies

J C Brocklehurst

First we must define an advanced (or developed) society. While most people understand what is meant by this very vague and perhaps contentious phrase, it is one that is more easily understood than defined. Basically it is an industrial society. Sometimes it is called a 'western' society, but this is a misnomer. Perhaps it might be defined as *a society in which at least 10% of the population is aged 65 or over* and for the present purposes this would be the most useful definition, for it is a definition which immediately encompasses one of the great problems of advanced societies—and the problem with which this book is concerned. A comparison of life expectancy in a representative group of countries sets this definition in a world context (Table 1.1).

One of the most important humanitarian advances brought about in the last hundred years has been the development of 'western' medicine and surgery to the point where death from disease during childhood or middle life, which used to be be the common fate of most people, has now become the exception. The majority of deaths (other than those due to trauma) occur as a result of a disease after the age of 65. Above all, the antibiotics and chemotherapeutic drugs have brought about this incredible change in the life and health of our people. Other factors such as improved surgical techniques, replacement and antimitotic drugs, improved diet and general hygiene of society and, in particular, preventative innoculation, have all played their part.

Now we have an ageing society and unfortunately medical progress in the prevention or cure of chronic disease lags far behind its fantastic

Table 1.1 Life expectancy at birth. The figures in this Table are derived from calculation by Rhee, H. A. (1974). *Human Aging and Retirement*, and are based on figures obtained through the mid-1960s.

	Female	*Male*	*Difference (F–M)*
Europe			
Northern	74.10	69.2	5.8
Western	74.2	68.2	6.0
Central	72.8	67.0	5.8
Eastern	72.1	67.0	5.1
Southern	71.10	67.0	4.10
All Europe	73.2	67.8	5.6
Canada	75.2	68.10	6.4
Japan	74.4	69.1	5.3
Australia	74.2	67.11	6.3
Uruguay	71.7	65.6	6.1
Chile	59.11	54.5	5.4
Pakistan	48.10	53.8	-5.0
India	44.7	41.11	2.8
Nigeria	36.8	37.2	-0.4
		Female & Male	
Ethiopia, Yemen and Mali		35	
Nepal		35–38	
Guinea		26–28	

(All figures in years and months)

success in relation to acute and infective disease. Above all, the 'western' scourge of atherosclerosis and its attendant pleomorphic morbidity in the elderly has yet to yield its secrets.

Old age, therefore (a stage which we will all reach), is more likely to be associated with disease and disability than any other period in the life span. It follows that medical problems of old age should command high priority in resource expenditure if a society wishes not only to provide for its older members as each of us would be provided for, but also if it is to avoid the economic burden of a vast mass of disabled and dependent old people.

The subsequent chapters in this book describe how a number of advanced nations are dealing with this late 20th Century problem. While the problem is the same in each country and while there is a common core in the approach which has been adopted, there are also the widest variations and an immediate objection may be that the restriction of this study to six countries can at the best provide only a patchy microcosm of the way in which the problem is being dealt with universally. The nations that are the subjects of this book are Australia, Great Britain, Holland, Sweden, USA and the USSR. Clearly the findings may have been different if instead one had looked at France. Norway, Spain, Brazil and Italy—or any other of the advanced societies—and this is acknowledged. Those that have been chosen, however, do tend to have a more developed system of medical care for the elderly than a number of other advanced societies and they do encompass a number of very different approaches to national administration and are, therefore, useful to compare.

The structure of each of the six chapters is different. The emphasis is on different aspects of medical care for the elderly, although in each case the central description of the present situation covers the same ground. In other ways, however, the chapters complement each other. Thus the whole background to demography, morbidity and mortality in old age is dealt with in detail only by Dr van Zonneveld in relation to Holland. The situation that he describes, however, is common to all six countries with relatively minor variations. Again, varying emphasis has been put on the history of the development of care for old people in the different countries, with the most detail in relation to Great Britain. Once more it is likely (at least up to the beginning of the 20th Century) that the historical development of care has been similar in the six countries. Indeed, until the present century the old as a group were so small as not to form a major area of concern. Many of them, unfortunately, had a common cause with the poor (even if they had not been impoverished throughout their whole lives) and the fear of the workhouse—a very understandable fear in 19th Century England—was mirrored in the other countries. The development of alms-houses too and the part played by charity was common.

Dr Revutskaya's description of the USSR brings out particularly the preventive aspects of medical care of old people and while prevention of illness (and its early ascertainment) receives mention in several of the chapters, the particular emphasis on physical culture described by Dr Revutskaya is probably less typical of other countries.

The emergence of a specialty of geriatric medicine (in Sweden called long-term care) has so far become a reality in only two of the six nations described and Great Britain has the distinction of leading in this field by about a quarter of a century. This specialty is, therefore, described in some detail in the chapter on Great Britain and leads logically to some consideration of medical education in relation to care of the elderly.

The method of financing services has most impact on individual people if it involves heavy expenditure at the time when illness attacks. Finance also may be a disincentive to development if payment for different categories of care comes from different sources. These implications of finance are most relevant (and are dealt with at greatest length) in relation to Australia and the USA.

British readers will find some difficulty with the term 'nursing-home' which has a different connotation in Great Britain to the other countries; in fact, terminology inevitably provides a difficulty in a book of this kind, and the different types of care described have been defined in the various chapters as far as seemed reasonable. In general, a nursing-home in all the countries is a place providing intermediate or long-stay care. In some instances, nursing-homes are privately financed and in other instances financed and owned by the state.

Finally, social care cannot be divorced from medical care in the field of old age. This, however, is such a huge topic on its own that generally the evolution and present situation in relation to pensions and social security arrangements have not been described, although various social services which have a bearing on medical care of old people have.

A synthesis is attempted in the final chapter. Clearly there are lessons to be learned from the similarities and from the differences inherent in the different systems of medical care. While a book of this type may be of interest in its general descriptions and while the reader will no doubt make his own comparisons and attempt to draw his own conclusions, it would be incomplete without some discussion of the common difficulties and perhaps the unique solutions. What will certainly emerge is that nowhere is medical care for old people as good as it should or could be. However, since all advanced societies have a common problem of aging and a basically similar approach to life, it is likely that a common pattern will begin to emerge sooner or later in what will be judged the optimum way ahead.

CHAPTER TWO

Great Britain

J C Brocklehurst

HISTORY

As in most European countries, medical care in Great Britain began with the church and the gradual development of infirmaries within its monasteries. Both St Thomas' and St Bartholomew's hospitals in London came into being in this way and both of these were closed in 1540 during the suppression of the monasteries by Henry VIII. However, the subsequent accumulation of the sick and lame in London streets created the obvious need for alternative accommodation and St Bartholomew's was re-opened in 1547 to be run by the Lord Mayor of London. Ten years later, St Thomas' was re-opened in a collective charter of the Royal Hospitals which included Christ's Hospital (for orphaned children), Bethlehem (for the lunatic poor) and Bridewell (for idle rogues).

Even at that early stage in the history of hospital care, official advice was given that patients whose illness was thought to be incurable should not be admitted to the Royal Hospitals and instead, out-houses were established outside London to accommodate the chronic sick.

The next stage, and perhaps the first real move towards care of the elderly was the passing of the Poor Relief Act of 1601 (the 43rd of Elizabeth) which required each parish to provide for the poor by levying a rate on all occupiers of property within the parish. The overseer of the poor was appointed in each parish to collect the rate and to see that it was spent on the relief of the aged and infirm poor, the binding apprentice of pauper children and the provision of some form of work for the able-bodied poor. This was followed in 1662 by the Act of Settlement which allowed parish overseers to return to their own parish 'settlement' people who had arrived within a parish to which they did not legally belong.

These two Acts formed the basis of the old Poor Law and in it the fortunes of the old were firmly bound up with those of the lame, the deaf and the blind (the chronic sick) and with the poor.

Gradually the church-wardens and overseers acquired workhouses in which to provide 'indoor' rather than 'outdoor' relief. Many of these became the seat of abuse and oppression and an attempt was made in 1782 to separate the elderly and disabled from the poor, the former group to be looked after in the workhouse, the latter given outdoor relief.

The rigours of life in the workhouse, however, were reinforced following the Royal Commission on the Poor Laws which was appointed in 1832 and reported in 1834. This report enshrined the principle of 'lesser eligibility' by which it was laid down that life in the workhouse should be made less attractive than the least attractive existence which the unfortunate person was likely to encounter in the slums of industrial 19th-Century England.

> 'The first and most essential of all conditions, a principle which we find universally admitted, even by those whose practice is at variance with it, is that, his situation on the whole shall not be made really or apparently so eligible as, the situation of the independent labourer of the lowest class'.

The general principle was that relief would only be given to paupers through their admission to the workhouse.

> 'All relief whatever to able-bodied persons or to their families, otherwise than in well regulated workhouses . . . shall be declared unlawful and shall cease'.

(Royal Commission on the Poor Laws Report 1834)

It was suggested that the unhappy involvement of the aged and chronic sick in this system should be mitigated wherever possible by special arrangements for them. Indeed, the elderly were divided into those of 'good report' for whom it was felt some special arrangements were appropriate and the 'aged poor of bad conduct'—for whom the workhouse remained a suitable place.

> 'For old men and women of this kind the general mixed workhouse with its stigma of pauperism, its dull routine, its exaction of such work

as its inmates can perform, and its deterrent regulations seems a fitting place in which to end a misspent life'.

(Minority report, the Royal Commission on the Poor Laws, 1834)

Workhouses gradually developed infirmaries when it became clear that special accommodation was needed for those who were ill. The infirmaries very soon became peopled with the aged and chronic sick and they themselves became the subject of indignant comment from a number of reformers. For instance, a medical officer to the Huddersfield Union Workhouse described the infirmary in July 1848 as follows:

'. . . the hospital was extremely filthy. The floors were filthy. I don't think they had been washed down throughout the hospital from the time of its being opened; marks of uncleanliness presented themselves nearly everywhere; cobwebs hung from the ceilings; the coverings of the beds were deficient, mere rags some of them; some of the blankets would hardly hold together if you would shake them'.

As a result of this and other reports, the *Lancet* set up in 1865 a team of three doctors to investigate this aspect of hospital care and they produced the Lancet Sanitary Commission for Investigating the State of the Infirmaries of Workhouses, Report 1866.

The *Lancet* team pointed out that not only the infirmaries, but the majority of the accommodation in many of the workhouses was occupied by sufferers from chronic disease. They described these as follows:

'The fate of the "infirm" inmates of crowded workhouses is lamentable in the extreme; they lead a life which would be like that of a vegetable, were it not that it preserves the doubtful privilege of sensibility to pain and mental misery. They are regarded by the officials connected with the establishment as an anomalous but unavoidable nuisance'.

The *Lancet* report then strikes a rational and indeed a modern note when it refers to the fate of a tradesman who because of chronic cough and a hard winter became bankrupt and eventually had to enter the workhouse, where he was assigned to the infirm ward to become one of hundreds of similar cases. The *Lancet* says:

'Now in this condition of infirm health the broken down tradesman may go on for years and, as such, is a consumer of the rates, a burden on the State at a cost per week we leave to be cast up by an official. If, as we assert ought to be the case, all the infirm were medically treated, there would be a very large percentage of recovery, and consequently, as before stated, an important saving of the rates'.

The extent to which the aged and chronic sick constituted the inhabitants of workhouses may be deduced from the following figures for the London Metropolitan Workhouses in January 1869:

6000 ordinary sick including lying-in
5000 old and infirm requiring medical care
1700 imbeciles
2400 children
10 500 healthy old people
3000 able-bodied people (Hodgkinson, 1967)

This in a total population of three million.

Gradually (and partly with the assistance of Florence Nightingale) trained nurses were introduced to the staff of the workhouse infirmary. The Metropolitan Poor Act of 1867 proposed that four or five unions should jointly build asylums for the general sick poor. In fact, two of these were built which along with the remaining poor law infirmaries continued to provide the majority of care for ill and disabled old people until the introduction of the National Health Service in 1948.

The British hospital scene, of course, throughout the 18th and 19th Centuries included two other types of hospitals. First, there were added to the Royal Hospitals a series of County Hospitals and major infirmaries, built as a result of voluntary subscriptions, in the main cities. These became the seat of the study and practice of medicine and as with the Royal Hospitals their emphasis was on acute disease and indeed they specifically excluded the aged and chronic sick.

The third group of hospitals were truly State Hospitals and included a large number of isolation hospitals for infectious fevers built in the second half of the 19th Century, institutions for tuberculosis built at the beginning of the 20th Century and large mental hospitals of anything beyond 2000 beds. Public General Hospitals were also built, many of them adjoining workhouses. They were generally required to take in all those in need of care. These hospitals gradually lost the stigma of their workhouse origin and attachment and became a second system of general hospitals set against the voluntary hospitals. Because they were state-owned and could not, therefore, be selective, they gradually accumulated the large numbers of aged and chronic sick who were prevented from admission to the voluntary hospitals and who were then able to escape direct admission to the workhouse infirmary *via* the workhouse itself. In 1948 77 000 beds in voluntary hospitals and 13 000 beds in public institutions were taken over by the National Health Service.

It was in these latter beds that the newly emerging specialty of geriatric medicine appeared in the late 1930s. The person who is generally regarded as the first pioneer in geriatric medicine is the late Dr Marjorie Warren who, while a Deputy Medical Superintendent at the West Middlesex Hospital in London (a public hospital), took charge of the associated workhouse infirmary. She realised, totally ahead of her time, that the infirmary contained large numbers of patients who were inadequately diagnosed and improperly treated, many of whom had been admitted for episodes of acute disease such as respiratory infection against a background of chronic disability and others who were admitted with increasing disability due to strokes and other chronic disorders. Once they had been admitted, medical attention was scanty and while nursing was of a high standard, many became permanently bedfast because the possibility of recovery was not recognised and there was indeed a total absence of facilities for rehabilitation. Dr Warren soon realised that the normal methods of medical examination and investigation if properly applied and followed by appropriate treatment, including physical treatment, could allow the majority of permanently bedfast patients to get up from their beds and in many cases to walk again and to be able to leave the infirmary. So, gradually, the whole face of treatment for chronic disease changed and with it changes in the character of the infirmaries had to follow. Because of the prejudices entrenched in tradition these changes were not made without a great deal of conflict. The early pioneers in geriatrics had great difficulty even in obtaining chairs for their patients to sit on and slippers and dressing gowns for them to wear.

Dr Warren was an early advocate of specialisation in geriatrics. She suggested that 'chronic sick' patients should be classified and looked after by different types of doctors as follows:

Paediatricians
General Physicians
Geriatricians
Psychiatrists
Tuberculosis Physicians

She felt that hospitals for the chronic sick should be replaced whenever possible.

'In the hospital for the chronic sick, both staff and patients are isolated from the more academic atmosphere of the General Hospital. Under such conditions indolence is likely to occur from lack of facilities which exist in the General Hospital, but which are too costly to justify duplication'.

(Warren, 1949)

Life in the workhouse infirmary at the time of the inception of the National Health Service has been well-described by Andrews (1971). Andrews described the rows of beds in which patients lay perhaps for years on end, well-nursed but with no prospect of recovery and no incentive to communicate even with the unfortunate individuals in the beds on each side.

...'rows of tidy beds with bedclothes carefully tucked in, producing the foot deformities so well-known to the early geriatric physicians. Bed rest led to protein depletion with muscle wasting, bony rarefaction and contractures. More important, it led to a state of apathy or contentment which was later to prove the mortal enemy of rehabilitation. The patient who had been three years in bed was usually to be classed as irremediable'.

THE SPECIALTY OF GERIATRIC MEDICINE

The National Health Service Act of 1946 made it possible, within a state service, to promote a new medical specialty. Following the inception of the National Health Service, the first publicly advertised appointment as *Geriatric Physician* was to Barncoose Hospital in Cornwall. This was rapidly followed by other similar appointments and throughout the subsequent twenty-five years almost 300 consultants in geriatric medicine were appointed in the United Kingdom. The majority of these were 'first generation' consultants in geriatrics and it is only within the last few years that retirement of these first-generation consultants has led to the appointment of second-generation specialists. In addition, an increasing number of departments have now a second consultant and in some cases a third and fourth.

The work which the first-generation consultants had to undertake was much the same and mirrored the pioneer work that has been described above undertaken by Dr Majorie Warren. Administrative arrangements within the National Health Service were based on Regional Hospital Boards (of which there were fourteen in England, one in Wales, four in Scotland and one in Northern Ireland). In each of these, hospitals were grouped together in Hospital Management Groups, each group being managed by a Hospital Management Committee composed principally of appointed (not elected) laymen and doctors.

Hospital groups served populations of generally between a quarter and half a million people and the Hospital Management Committee would have responsibility for all the hospitals within the group; a common secretariat would be developed and while many consultants were in contract to more than one group, in geriatric medicine it was more common for a consultant to be appointed to develop the service for one hospital group. This meant, nevertheless, that he was given charge of beds very often in five, six or more different hospitals. These beds were usually in hospital wards built for quite different purposes which were no longer required for those purposes. He might thus have some wards in a general hospital, others in a former infectious diseases hospital, in a former sanitorium, in an old workhouse infirmary and possibly in a number of cottage hospitals. All these beds, of course, would be filled with old people and there would be every chance that a waiting list of a hundred or more, created on a purely administrative basis, awaited his arrival.

He had to determine, therefore, how he would use the beds in the various hospitals to weld them into a unit. The pattern that evolved generally throughout the country was one of three levels of in-patient care—an early form of progressive patient care. Some beds, and particularly those that might be available in a general hospital, would be used as the *acute beds* for the majority of the admissions to the department. This would become the acute ward (or assessment ward as it was often called) and here the initial investigation to make a comprehensive diagnosis and the initiation of treatment was made and decisions taken as to the patient's likely future, having in mind both the social and medical implications of his illness.

The second eschalon of wards would be designated *rehabilitation wards* and would be situated in the most favourable location for obtaining services of occupational therapists and physiotherapists.

The third group of wards would be used for the *long-term care* of patients who were not going to leave the hospital and these would, with advantage, be situated in geographically different parts of the area where they might be near to the localities where the patients had their roots.

The first task that the newly appointed consultant would have to undertake would be, like Majorie Warren, to examine all the patients occupying the beds he had taken over, and to determine to what extent they could be rehabilitated and restored to an independent life in the community. This process occupied the first few months of the newly-appointed consultant's career and it was often a few years before the department began to achieve a turnover as the effect of exclusion of patients who could be maintained independently in other ways, had its impact.

The second task which the new consultant would have to undertake would be a review of the waiting list. To do this he would visit all the patients on the waiting list, in their own homes. Only by this means could the waiting list become meaningful. Some estimate could be made of the real need for admission and the urgency with which admission must be accomplished. Alternative methods of care, either by short-stay pre-arranged admission, by attendance as an out-patient, or possibly by admission to an old person's home, would wherever possible be implemented.

Therefore, at an early stage two important principles of geriatric practice were established—that of assessment visiting before the admission of patients into hospital and that of progressive patient care.

In addition to coping with an existing waiting list the pre-admission assessment visit allowed the geriatrician to obtain a much more complete picture of his patient and the patient's social background. In addition, the history might be obtained from a relative or neighbour in cases where it was unobtainable from the patient himself because of deafness, dysphasia, or mental disorder. The pre-admission assessment visit also allowed a discussion with relatives as to the proposed management of the case and particularly that their expectation of hospital admission should not be interpreted as final and irrevocable committal to the hospital. Gradually the remedial and supportive aspects of the geriatric hospital department emerged and the practice of pre-admission assessment visiting made a great contribution to this.

DEMOGRAPHY

The national census of 1971

The population of the United Kingdom like that of all other Western societies is showing an accelerating trend towards increase in the proportion of the very old. Table 2.1 indicates the increase in the proportion of population in different age groups predicted in the twenty years from 1971 to 1991. While there will be an overall increase of 8.25% the increase of the over 65s will be almost double that; the increase of the over 75s almost quadruple this figure. The increase in the 85s and over is more than five times that for the population as a whole, showing an increase of 42%. As is to be expected, it is the very old who figure most largely among the ranks of the disabled.

Table 2.1 Population increase—different age groups 1971-1991 (United Kingdom—No. in thousands) (*From Population Projections* (1972) No. 2 1971-2011 by courtesy of HMSO)

		1971	*1991*	*% Increase*
All	M	27 081	29 523	
Ages	F	28 587	30 740	
	Total	55 668	60 263	8.25
65+	M	2757	3238	
	F	4446	5113	
	Total	7203	8351	15.94
75+	M	804	1124	
	F	1718	2340	
	Total	2522	3464	37.35
85+	M	121	159	
	F	344	503	
	Total	465	662	42.37

Table 2.2 indicates the rate of disability in different age groups. It shows that while approximately 2% of the population may be described as disabled, the vast majority of disabled are also aged 75 years or over. These figures relate to physical disability. If we look at figures for mental disorder, we may take as most typical those from a survey carried out in Newcastle which indicated that 6% of the elderly population were suffering from moderate or marked dementia and more than twice this number were suffering from mild dementia (Roth *et al.,* 1964).

Table 2.2 The prevalence of disability in Great Britain and its relationship to people over the age of seventy-five. (From Harris, A. I. (1971), by courtesy of HMSO)

	Disabled	*Age 75+*	*% Aged 75+*
Very severely handicapped (needing special care)	157 000	115 000	73
Severely handicapped (needing considerable support)	356 000	227 000	64
Appreciably handicapped (needing some support)	616 000	389 000	63
Total disabled	1 129 000	731 000	64
Total population	54 000 000	2 500 000	

Table 2.3 indicates the disposition of people aged 65 and over between domiciliary and institutional care in 1962. This survey carried out by Townsend and Wedderburn (1965) was part of the cross-national survey published in detail in the book, *Old People in Three Industrial Societies,*

Table 2.3 Estimated number of persons aged sixty-five and over living in different types of accommodation: Britain, Mid-1962 (From Townsend and Wedderburn (1965), by courtesy of Bell)

Type of accommodation	*Persons aged 65 or over*		
	Number	*%*	
1. Residential homes	105 000	1.7	4.5
2. Psychiatric hospitals and nursing-homes	60 000	1.0	
3. Other hospitals and nursing homes	115 000	1.8	
4. Hotels, boarding houses, hostels, common lodging houses, etc.	95 000	1.5	95.5
5. Private households	5 825 000	94.0	
Total	62 000 000	100.0	

(Shanus, 1968). It showed at that time that 4.5% of the elderly population of Great Britain were living in institutions and that all the others were living either in their own or their children's homes or else in private hotels, boarding houses, etc. Of the 4.5% living in institutions, 1.7% were in residential homes and 2.8% in hospitals and nursing-homes.

Table 2.4 indicates the distribution of hospitalised elderly people

Table 2.4 Beds occupied by patients aged sixty-five and over (England and Wales 1965) (one third of all hospital beds)

% of beds in specialty occupied by patients 65+	*Department*	*Distribution of patients 65+*
88%	Geriatrics/chronic sick	34.0%
43%	General medicine	10.0%
28%	Other general hospital departments	20.0%
39%	Psychiatric	36.0%
36%	Total	100.0%

among the different hospital departments, showing that while the largest proportion of patients in geriatric wards are old people (as would be expected), medical and surgical wards also carry a large proportion of elderly people, among their in-patients. There is no doubt that the inevitable trend over the rest of the 20th Century will be for in-patients in all general hospital wards to fall more and more into the old age groups.

Table 2.5 indicates the number of beds available for geriatric patients and those requiring long-term care, together with the turn-over per bed and new out-patient attendances from 1959 to 1971. During these twelve years the turn-over per bed rose by 26% and the new out-patient attendances more than trebled.

This is the backcloth against which must be viewed the present arrangements for the elderly and future trends in their care.

Table 2.5 Geriatrics and chronic sick—bed provision and usage. (England and Wales—No. in thousands) (From *Health and Personal Social Services Statistics* (1972), by courtesy of HMSO)

	1949	*1959*	*1964*	*1969*	*1971*
Beds available		57	58	59	61
Deaths and discharges	81	135	157	179	187
Turnover/bed		2.4	2.7	3:0	3.1
Out-patients New attendances		9	16	25	29

GERIATRIC PRACTICE

In many areas the pre-admission assessment visit remains a cardinal principle of geriatric practice, although some consultants now prefer to admit all patients immediately on demand from general practitioners. This allows a higher proportion of medical emergencies in the elderly to be dealt with by the geriatric department and this goal has always been a very appealing one to geriatricians. On the other hand, pre-admission assessment visits allow a more balanced decision to be made and is certainly an invaluable system during a consultant's first few years in his area, encouraging him to become intimately familiar with the various patterns of housing and social care. He sees the problems at first hand in their natural setting.

The pre-admission assessment visit is one initiated by the hospital as one way of dealing with requests for admission by general practitioners. This has to be distinguished from the domiciliary consultation in which advice is requested by a family doctor from a consultant geriatrician either on the clinical management of a patient or on the medico-social problems. This visit is initiated by the general practitioner and not by the hospital doctor and it attracts an individual fee for the consultant which does not apply to the pre-admission assessment visit.

The different elements of progressive patient care which have now become the fairly standard setting for geriatric medicine may well be illustrated by quoting the figures for one large geriatric department in South Manchester. These are illustrated in the accompanying diagrams.

The acute geriatric ward (Figure 2.1) receives its patients from their

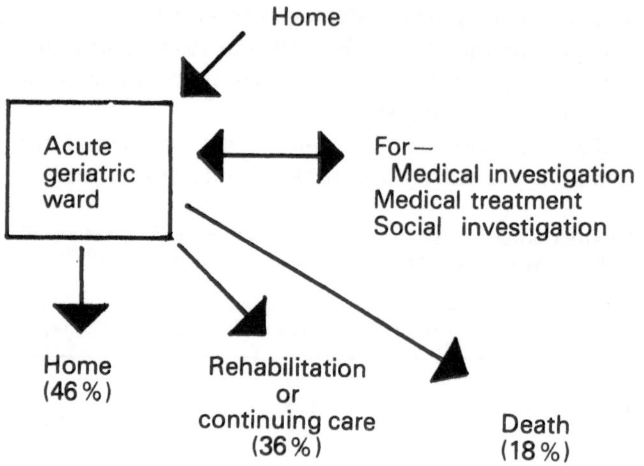

Figure 2.1 The acute geriatric ward

own homes or from old people's homes and 46% of them return home, 36% to rehabilitation or continuing care wards and 18% die. The average length of stay is two to three weeks and the emphasis is entirely that of an acute general ward, that is, medical investigation and treatment and social investigation with assessment of the patient's future.

The rehabilitation ward (Figure 2.2) receives most of its patients from the acute geriatric ward but also some from medical, surgical and orthopaedic wards (they have been investigated and now require physical treatment.) These are particularly patients with stroke, arthritis, Parkinsonism and fracture of the femur. The length of stay is two to three months. About 57% then return either home or to an old people's home, 16% die and 27% move on to the continuing care or long-stay wards.

Treatment in the rehabilitation wards is by the rehabilitation team, consisting of physician, nurse, social worker, occupational therapist, physiotherapist and speech therapist. Patients are reviewed at weekly case-conferences and all the members of the team should be involved in this review. The accent throughout is on physical, social and mental rehabilitation. The nursing staff are careful to get away from the protectiveness which is so much a part of a nurse's training. The nursing duties involve a considerable degree of overlap with the work of the therapists.

Continuing care wards (or long-stay wards) (Figure 2.3) receive most of

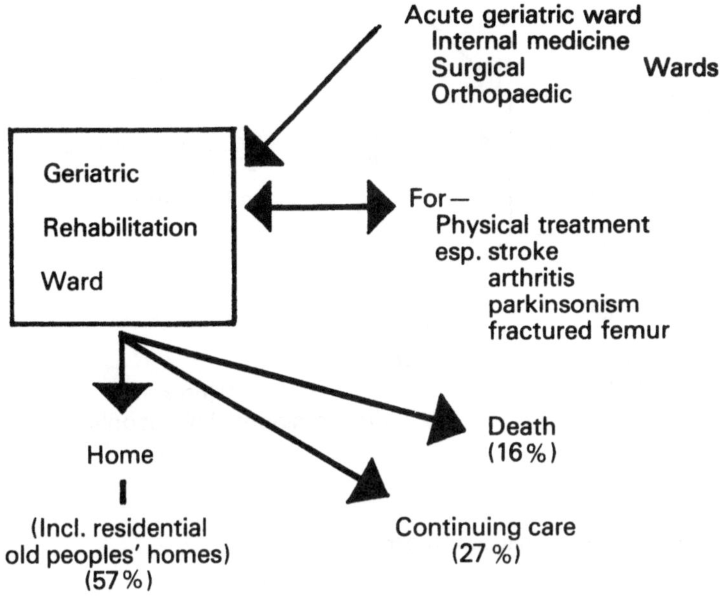

Figure 2.2 The rehabilitation geriatric ward

their patients from the rehabilitation wards when it becomes apparent that the patient is not going to achieve the necessary physical or mental independence to go home or live in an old persons' home. In some cases this may be apparent without a preliminary period of rehabilitation and such patients are admitted directly from other acute wards.

In continuing care wards there is always a proportion of patients who will recover slowly but about 90% of the patients remain there until death. The average length of stay is two to three years. The continuing care ward, therefore, is clearly the patient's home for the remainder of his life and while some patients will be there for only a few months others will live for five, ten and even fifteen years. The need for properly purpose-built accommodation for patients of this type is, therefore, very apparent. (Quality of care, of course, does not always match the quality of the buildings.) In Great Britain almost no purpose-built long-stay accommodation for elderly people as yet exists and indeed many such people are still housed in workhouse infirmaries built in the middle of the 19th Century.

Long-stay care—the provision of a home—should mean the provision

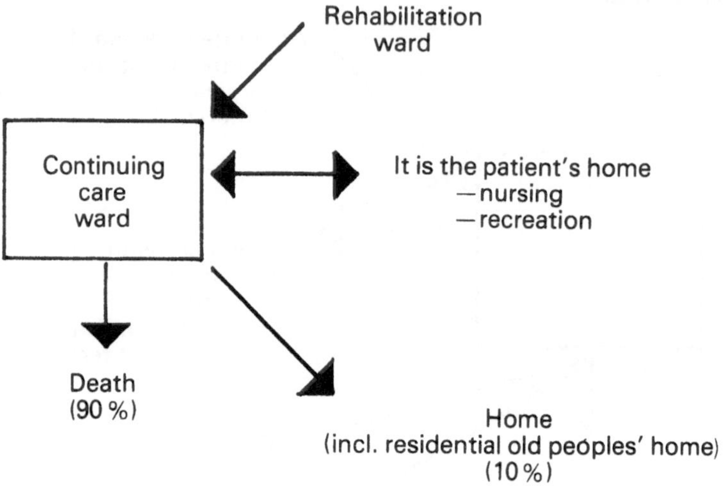

Figure 2.3 The continuing care geriatric ward

of privacy and at the same time facilities for creative and recreational activities to make life worth living. It would seem reasonable, therefore, that these wards should provide single rooms for the majority of patients, and that there should be a proper suite of dining room, lounge and recreation rooms, including an art studio and access to a garden. Most of these patients may move around in wheelchairs and it is only the last few weeks of their lives that most old people become bedfast.

That such a vision of long-stay care is neither modern nor revolutionary may be indicated by the following quotation from the *British Medical Journal* of 1856.

> 'At Bethlehem Hospital there are some convalescent wards which fill with pleasure the mind of the philanthropic physician. Here the patient not only finds cheerful, light literature and the current newpapers but the windows are fitted up with vivaria, ferneries and cages full of birds and the smaller animals. It is impossible to estimate too highly the value of these little aids to pass the vacant hours, yet we venture to say that in ninety-nine cases out of one hundred the members of the Hospital Board who would propose the introduction of such cheap amusements as these for the patients would be laughed at'.

The contrast between this approach to long-stay care and the all too common present situation was well-described by Halliburton and Wright (1973).

In America the provision of single rooms although by no means universal is much more accepted than in Great Britain. In this country, however, we are seeing a movement to introduce professionally trained tutors from local authority Colleges of Further Education to teach painting, crafts, music appreciation and so on (Poulden, 1971; Bright, 1972). The latent creative potential which has been realized in large numbers of very old people as a result of the provision of these facilities is one of the marvels of geriatric medicine. In addition to these activities, the formation of patient's clubs, the involvement of volunteers and some participation in community activities, are all aspects of long-stay geriatric care for which the geriatrician has a responsibility and in which he is only now beginning to realise the role that he should be playing.

The geriatric day hospital is a logical development of progessive patient care and the majority of geriatric departments in Great Britain now include a day hospital. The day hospital movement had its origins in the Soviet Union in the 1930s with day hospitals for psychiatric patients; psychiatric day hospitals were the first in the field in the United Kingdom. The early development of day hospitals has been well-described by Farndale (1961) and more recently the position has been reviewed by Brocklehurst (1970). The first purpose-built day hospital in the United Kingdom was Cowley Road Hospital, Oxford, opened in 1958. Now the Department of Health and Social Security lays down a norm of two day-hospital places to every 1000 of the population aged 65 and over (and in addition two psycho-geriatric day-hospital places per 1000 people aged 65 and over).

The geriatric day hospital is an attempt to dissociate the hotel aspects of geriatric in-patient care from the therapeutic aspect. It appreciates that many patients remain in hospital when they could equally well be living at home at nights and over the weekends and coming to the hospital only in the day-time for treatment. Not only are there advantages to patients themselves in getting home at such an early stage of their illness, but in a situation where staff are in increasingly short supply it provides for an economic deployment of nurses.

The day hospital is generally open five days a week and almost all patients come by ambulance provided by the National Health Service. Only gradually are appropriate vehicles being provided by the ambulance service and in many areas the multipurpose vehicles (which can be used both for emergencies and also for bringing sitting patients to hospitals) are still in use. The importance of properly designed ambulance vehicles for patients coming to geriatric day hospitals is the same as that of the purpose-designed provision for in-patients. The vehicle should ideally carry eight people, who should be safe and comfortably seated in a warm temperature. The vehicle should provide good vision since some of the patients will spend upwards of an hour on a journey. While this could be exhausting, if the vehicle is comfortable and provides good vision, it will be an enjoyable experience for the elderly patient for whom it almost certainly marks the only time he ever leaves his own home. Day hospitals, of course, are particularly exposed to industrial disputes involving ambulance crews. These have not been an uncommon part of the British scene over the last few years. (The effect of such a dispute has been described by Prinsley, 1971.)

The principal diagnosis of patients attending a group of day hospitals in the south-east of England is shown in Table 2.6. The diagnosis itself,

Table 2.6 Principal diagnoses of patients attending geriatric day hospitals (From Brocklehurst (1970), by courtesy of King Edward's Hospital Fund for London)

Arthritis or fractured femur	30%
Stroke	30%
Cerebral arteriosclerosis, dementia, Parkinsonism, other diseases of the central nervous system	22%
Depression	4%
Other disease	14%

however, does not explain the reason why the patient is attending the day hospital. This is better appreciated if expressed in terms of (*a*) rehabilitation (*b*) maintenance treatment (*c*) social care and (*d*) medical and nursing procedures. These are the reasons why patients attend day hospitals. A patient with the diagnosis of stroke, for example, might be attending for any one of these reasons.

It is important that the clinician asks himself, 'Why is this patient attending the day hospital?' and answers the question satisfactorily, since this allows a much more precise use of facilities which may otherwise be carelessly used and thus become expensive. Table 2.7 shows the reason for attendance among the same group of patients referred to in Table 2.6. Those coming for rehabilitation may either leave hospital at

Table 2.7 Reasons for attending a geriatric day hospital (From Brocklehurst (1970), by courtesy of King Edward's Hospital Fund for London)

Rehabilitation	27%
Physical maintenance	42%
Social reasons	26%
Others	5%

an earlier stage than might otherwise be possible or else may come for this form of treatment without ever having to be admitted to hospital at all.

The label 'maintenance treatment' registers the fact that most disease in old age is incurable. Rehabilitation will restore maximal independence Once rehabilitation is ended, if the patient is cut off entirely from physical therapy he will very often deteriorate to such a point that the benefit received from a prolonged course of hospital treatment may be entirely lost. Attendance at a day hospital one day a week may avert this situation.

Patients who come for social reasons are those who because of their physical disability are isolated. For them the opportunity to join with other elderly people in a stimulating social environment has obvious humanitarian and preventive aspects. Such patients may come one day a week to the day hospital; sometimes a physically disabled patient who needs constant attention from relatives may remain at home even if the relatives have to work for their living, provided he may be looked after in the day time at the day hospital. Such care is provided for patients who are so disabled that they need assistance of nurses and who for this reason could not be looked after in local authority Social Day Centres.

Patients may attend for medical and nursing procedures, including the observation and supervision of incontinence and day-long procedures, such as total dose iron infusions.

The geriatric day hospital is now firmly established as a form of geriatric care, but no critical study of the use of day hospitals has yet been produced. It is, of course, very difficult to show a 'before and after' situation when there may be so many variables other than the provision of a new day hospital. Similarly, a comparison of departments with and without day hospitals has its difficulties. Brocklehurst and Shergold (1969) attempted to make such a comparison in following-up patients discharged from two geriatric departments—one with and one without a geriatric day hospital.

The geriatric services and social class. It has been argued (Eckstein and Harvard, 1958) that medical services during the hundred years or so before the inauguration of the National Health Service developed to the advantage of the poor and to the disadvantage of the middle class. The rich, of course, were and continue to be able to afford to pay whatever is required. Whether or not this is true, there is little doubt that since the development of the Health Service many people of social class 2 have opted for treatment in private nursing-homes rather than in National Health Service hospitals. Almost without exception, these nursing-homes are inferior in terms of medical care, nursing care and facilities for rehabilitation, but they still cushion part of the load of geriatric illness, particularly in the wealthier parts of the country.

THE PLACE OF THE GENERAL PRACTITIONER IN THE CARE OF THE ELDERLY

With the emergence of the National Health Service in 1948, general practitioners retained their status as independent contractors and for a fixed capitation fee they undertook to provide a medical service for those people living in the area of their practice who wished to register with them. Patients were free to register with the doctor of their choice and doctors to accept or reject patients to their list. The ceiling to the number of patients on the general practitioner's list was stated and has fluctuated from time to time. The present ceiling is 3500 for a single-handed practitioner. Special arrangements for group practices allow a larger list. General practitioners agree to provide medical examination and treatment for patients who report to them with illness, together with prescriptions for drugs and certification for insurance purposes. Patients have never made a direct payment at the time of consultation and in principle drugs and appliances (including spectacles) have been free, but from time to time, the patient may be requested to pay up to £5·43 for spectacles £10 for dentures or dental treatment and 20 pence per prescription. There have always been excluded groups and these include old age pensioners.

Since 1st October 1966 a special payment has been made to general practitioners for every person aged 65 and over on their practice lists. This was in recognition of the increased work-load generated by people of this age.

It is notable that the general practitioners' service is geared towards the treatment of illness which patients report and neither the capitation fee nor the additional weighting for elderly people is intended to provide any form of preventive examination or treatment nor any system for the finding of unreported illness. These have, however, been matters in which some general practitioners have taken a lead and a number of experimental schemes for the ascertainment of unreported illness (involving general practitioners and ancillary workers attached to their practices) have been undertaken in the last few years.

During the past twenty-five years general practice has developed towards the concept of group practice and most recently a number of these groups have been provided with special premises (which they rent) by local authorities. Additional financial arrangements were negotiated in 1966 by which government subsidies were paid for the secretarial staff and practice nurses and in some areas during the last five to ten years it has been the practice of Medical Officers of Health to deploy health visitors on their staff by attaching them to individual general practices, sometimes part-time but very often full-time. The function of the health visitor is dealt with below. Her traditional role has centred on mothers and young children. However, it has seemed appropriate to use her particular expertise in the search for unreported illness among old people and this has been eagerly seized upon in areas where this system has been developing.

With the development of group practices and health centres the majority of general practitioners have now evolved appointment systems and there has been a strong trend towards surgery (office) consultations and a discouragement of patients' expecting home visits. While this has been acceptable to most of the population, it presents problems for old people who may have difficulty in using telephones and to whom, indeed, telephones may be quite inaccessible and who also may have great difficulty in getting to the doctor's surgery.

The practice of the regular (social) visiting of chronically ill and elderly patients at monthly or two-monthly intervals has gradually been diminishing over the last few years. The value of such visits from a purely medical point of view was very arguable since usually no medical examination was performed and the visit was one of social contact, very often with the renewal of a prescription. It may well be argued that a consultation for a particular and newly arising illness is likely to be of more positive value, or if regular visits are to be carried out then these should be to a clear structure in which some definite form of medical examination is included which might involve, for instance, the collection of blood or urine.

There can be no doubt that the system of general practice provides a convenient and acceptable form of primary medical care and a recent survey (The General Medical Services: Report of a Joint Working Party, 1973) has indicated that patients are pleased with it. From the point of view of the old person, however, some of the limitations include the increasing use of deputising services for night and week-end work and particularly the tendency for renewal prescriptions to be issued on some occasions time and time again, without the patient being seen.

ASCERTAINMENT OF UNREPORTED ILLNESS

It is well known that old people frequently attribute symptoms of pain, lethargy, dysuria and many others, not to illness, but to the fact that they are getting old. That a large amount of remediable illness has thus never been treated because it has never been reported was demonstrated by Williamson and his colleagues (1964). Analysis of Williamson's findings shows that unreported illness may be divided into two broad categories. The first is those of the major systems (Figure 2.4) where perhaps a good deal of that which is unreported is also irremediable. The second, those of simpler disabilities (Figure 2.5) where a far higher proportion is

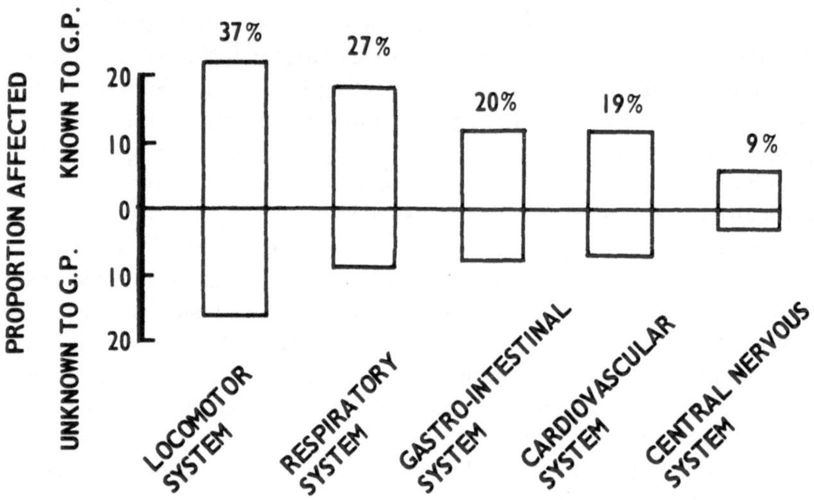

Figure 2.4 Incidence of disease in the elderly—major illnesses (Williamson *et al.*, 1964)

unknown to the doctor and yet far more is remediable. It is on the basis of these and other similar findings that the proposal to employ health visitors in making initial contact with elderly people has been developed. In some cases the health visitors have been trained to become expert at simple examinations of hearing and vision, looking at the teeth and feet, considering the mental state and evidence of heart failure, taking blood and urine samples and giving advice about social services. In other cases, the health visitors have simply taken a profile history and if the old person has been agreeable, then an appointment has been made for an examination by a doctor, either in a Health Centre or in a Health Clinic of the local authority and carried out either by a general practitioner or by a clinical public health doctor. That health visitors are as adept as

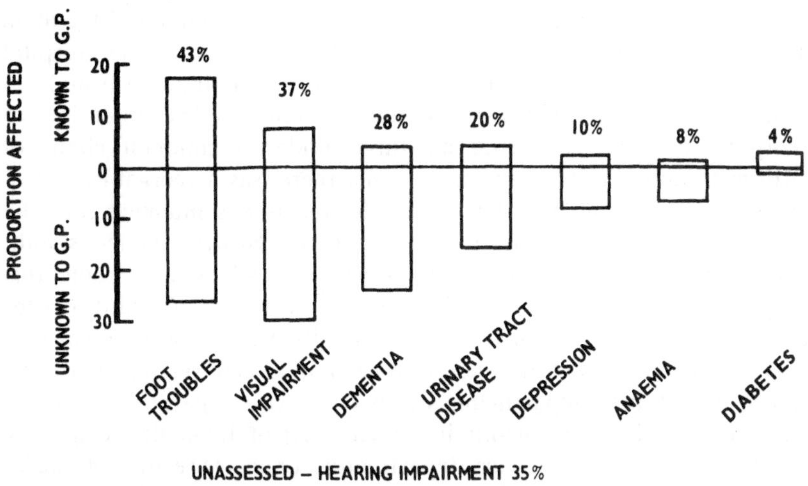

Figure 2.5 Incidence of disease in the elderly—minor illnesses (Williamson *et al.*, 1964)

clinicians in discovering these clinical signs has been demonstrated by Williamson *et al.* (1966).

Since each general practitioner is able to obtain an age/sex register of the patients on his list and since over 98% of all people in the United Kingdom are on the list of a general practitioner, he is clearly in the best position of anyone in the community to make contact with all the old people. Economically, this is impracticable at the present time and, therefore, it has been suggested that effort should be concentrated on high risk groups (such as the recently bereaved, the very old, those recently discharged from hospital and those who have not been seen by the general practitioner during the previous twelve months). The results of surveys of this type have been published (Lowther *et al.*, 1970; Williams *et al.*, 1972). Other systems of preventive care include those pioneered by Anderson and Cowan (1955) in Rutherglen, Scotland where a clinic has been set up for examination of old people who are not ill, but who feel it is desirable that they should have a medical examination.

THE REORGANISED NATIONAL HEALTH SERVICE

A complete reorganisation of the administration of the British National Health Service took place on 1st April 1974. The intention was to unify administration. Previously the Health Service had fallen into three main administrative groups—the General Practitioner Service, the Hospital Service and the Public Health Service (the last being financed from local sources; the other two from national sources). The intention of reorganisation was to bring all three under a common chain of administration. At about the same time, there was a reorganisation of local government areas in Great Britain and it was intended that the geographical units of administration of the Health Service should coincide with those of the new local government areas. On the whole, this has happened although there have been exceptions. A third matter which made this coincidence of administrative areas important was that in 1972 there was a total reorganisation of social services with the emergence of new departments of social service separated from the departments of public health in which most of them had originally developed. The social service departments, under Directors of Social Services, remain still as local authority departments with separate financing from the National Health Service (now financed entirely from central government departments). This is regrettable as far as areas of overlap between the two services are concerned, as in the care of mildly disabled old people, since both the Social Services and the National Health Service are likely to look to the other for a larger share of the expenditure and so these areas of neglect are likely to be perpetuated. It is hoped to overcome this in part by setting up within each administrative Health Service unit a 'Health Care Planning Team for the Elderly.' This is one of the multitudinous committees within the Health Service and it does provide an opportunity for unified planning for all medical and social services for old people in each area or district. Unfortunately, the Health Care Planning Teams have no executive responsibilities and time will tell whether or not they have any real contribution to make. The indications at present are that their decisions are more likely to be binding where they relate to the Hospital Service than where they relate to the Social Services.

The reorganised Health Service retains the regional structure of the old Health Service for the broad overall planning of policy under the following heads:

— the development of medical specialties
— deployment of medical manpower
— priorities of major building projects.

Within these fourteen regions, however, there are now ninety areas (the majority of which are divided into two or more districts). The district (or the area in the case of a single district area) is based on the district general hospital and is the focus for the total supply of medical services in that area or district. The unit of population served by a district is approximately 200 000-300 000. The district administration is responsible for all medical services including domiciliary and hospital nursing, therapy and general practice and all hospital departments. Forward planning within each district will be guided by a community physician (who is an epidemiologist and public health doctor), together with a small team of professional colleagues and a district administrator.

One additional provision which relates to care of the elderly is a body called a 'Community Health Council.' This is an elected body representing the consumers of the Health Service. Its members are elected both by voluntary bodies (such as Age Concern) and by local authorities. The Community Health Councils have a potential to monitor and guide the development of health care provision from the patients' point of view. As with all other innovations in the newly organised Health Service, it is as yet too early to assess the effect of the Community Health Councils. However, given wise leadership they could have an important impact in ensuring an equitable distribution of resources among all patients, including the elderly.

SOCIAL SERVICES

Social services are provided by the local authority. These developed as part of the department of the Medical Officer of Health and while in some areas they became a separate department, in most areas they remained a combined department until the Social Services Act of 1970 which was based on the findings of the Seebohm Committee. As a result of this legislation, entirely independent departments of Social Services were created in each local authority and these now have the responsibility for the whole range of social care, from problem families to residential care of the old people, including care of mentally handicapped, both at home and in institutions, the provision of home-helps, meals-on-wheels and so on. As might be expected, the development of entirely new departments of this type has not been without difficulty. The first year of such a department was characteristically described by Speed (1971). The emphasis of the Seebohm Committee was that social care should be family-centred and that social workers should be generic rather than specialised. They have become deployed in area teams at which level they have direct contact with their clients. The development of the Social Services has not been made easier by the reorganisation of local government in 1974—an attempt to rationalise the area boundaries and reduce the number of administrative units from fifty-eight to forty-five Metropolitan and non-Metropolitan Counties. These new Counties are now divided into 332 smaller administrative units (districts). The non-Metropolitan Counties and the Metropolitan Districts are the authorities running social service departments and they vary in unit population from about one million to about 30 000. With the reorganisation of the Health Service (see above) the Medical Social Workers, who are hospital based and who were formerly employees of the hospital service have now been added to the staff of the social service departments.

The principle now involved in the division between health and social services is that each shall act entirely independently and where medical services are required in the social field they shall be provided on secondment from the Area Health Authority; similarly where social services are required in the health field, they will be provided on secondment from the Social Services Department.

The most important social services which are concerned with the elderly are the home-help scheme (providing domestic help usually on an hourly basis and for which a fee is payable by the client), the provision of residential homes and of sheltered housing units (jointly with housing departments), the provision of day centres, luncheon clubs and sheltered workshops for the elderly (often in association with such workshops for the disabled), the provision of special fittings and fixtures in people's individual houses and of certain items of equipment for the disabled, (including walking aids, alternating-pressure mattresses, hoists) and the provision of domiciliary meals service (often in conjunction with the voluntary services—see below).

It may be appropriate to consider a few of these services in more detail.

Residential accommodation

This is provided under Part 3 of the National Assistance Act (1948) which required local authorities to provide residential accommodation for the elderly in need of care and attention which was not otherwise available.

In 1948 most residential care of this type was provided in former workhouses and, as with the Hospital Service, some still remains in upgraded 19th Century buildings. However, the social services have, in general, been far more successful in providing appropriate purpose-built accommodation than have the hospitals and the majority of old people's homes are now of this type. Townsend (1964) described the evolution of residential care up until that time and emphasised the need to develop short-term rather than long-term care. He drew attention to the enormous influence which the personality of the matron or manageress in charge has on the whole environment of the home and on the happiness of the lives of the elderly people living in it. Since then, attempts to provide training courses for staff of the homes have met with some success. Very often these are on a day-release basis. A small number of full-time courses have been set up.

Table 2.8 indicates the number of residents in residential homes from 1963 to 1969 including both State (local authority) homes and those run privately or by voluntary bodies. During this six year period there has been a 27% increase in this provision from 135 000 to 171 000.

Table 2.8 Number of persons in residential homes 1963-1969 (Great Britain—No. in thousands)

No. of residents		*1963*	*1966*	*1969*
Local authority residential homes	<65	11 518	12 058	12 536
	65+	88 489	97 939	111 041
Voluntary and private homes	65+	46 735	–	60 318
Total	65+	135 224	–	171 359 (27% increase)

The characteristics of the old people who live in these residential homes have changed greatly during the last twenty-five years. It is now generally realised that the majority of old people entering old people's homes will do so because of their inability to live independently, either because of physical or mental frailty. It is to be expected that very few physically (and/or mentally) fit old people will now opt to move into homes of this type in future and indeed it is increasingly difficult to provide them with such accommodation as the demands increase relentlessly.

The development of sheltered housing provides a much more satisfactory solution for most of these fitter old people. It allows them to have their own furniture and belongings, to organise their own lives and, at the same time, to have the security of an easily available warden. At the present time the provision of residential care is, on average, twenty-six places per 1000 people aged 65 and over of the general population; that this is well below the figure that is needed is indicated by the fact that most geriatric hospital departments have about 10% of their beds occupied by elderly people who have become fit to move into residential care and who are on the waiting list for such a transfer. That people should have to wait at this stage is regrettable (as indeed are all waiting lists) because it usually means that the optimum moment of transfer, after a period of rehabilitation, is lost and this is likely to add to the difficulty of these old people when they are eventually found a place in a residential home.

The frailty of old people in these homes has been referred to in a number of documents including the reports from Buckinghamshire and Hertfordshire County Councils (Buckingham County Council, 1973; Flowers and Parry, 1974).

Domiciliary meals service

Domiciliary meals (meals-on-wheels) were initiated by the Women's Voluntary Service during the last war. Through the subsequent quarter century they have, to a large extent, been provided by voluntary organisations, most particularly the WRVS. The meals are usually prepared in central kitchens, sometimes by volunteers and sometimes by paid cooks and then distributed in special vehicles to old people in their homes. The extent of this provision varies enormously from area to area, from one or two meals per person per week to a minimum of five and a maximum of seven per person per week. It is argued that if an old person really needs supplementary feeding of this type then this old person is probably quite unable to cook and that to maintain adequate nutrition, meals-on-wheels must be provided at least four days a week (see Exton-Smith and Stanton 1972). On this basis, where Social Services Departments have taken over the whole provision of these services, they usually strive to provide a minimum service of 5 days a week. The opposite viewpoint is that most old people can manage to provide for most of their dietary needs if some supplementation can be arranged and for this purpose meals twice a week are sufficient (see Davies *et al.*, 1974). There is no doubt that the majority of consumers in both cases are people who are capable of providing some food for themselves (Stanton, 1971). The argument is still developing. If meals are to be provided five or seven days a week then very close supervision will be required to see that when they are no longer needed they are withdrawn. It is obviously in the interests of old people themselves that they should be encouraged to attend a luncheon club or social day centre, adding to the purely nutritional value, the important fact that a meal is a social occasion.

Table 2.9 Cases attended by home-helps (England and Wales—No. in thousands) (From *Health and Personal Social Services Statistics* (1972), by courtesy of HMSO

	1963	*1967*	*1970*
Total cases attended	354.7	423.8	469.5
Persons aged 65+ attended	266.2	338.3	396.0
Persons 65+ attended per 1000 persons 65+ in the population	47.4	55.9	62.3

The Social Service Department also provides a home-help service. The home-help undertakes domestic work, shopping and sometimes the preparation of simple meals. This service plays a very important part in maintaining frail and disabled elderly people at home. A fee is payable but part or all of this is waived if the old person cannot afford it.

Table 2.9 indicates the increase in the total number of cases attended by home-helps from 1963 to 1970 and shows that among persons 65 and over this figure has risen from forty-seven per 1000 in 1963 to sixty-two per 1000 in 1970.

VOLUNTARY CARE

Voluntary care has always figured very largely in providing for the needs of more disabled citizens in the United Kingdom and this has been true no less for the elderly than for the blind, the deaf, the mentally handicapped and those suffering from various types of physical disability. The chief national organisation providing this type of care is Age Concern which was set up in 1940 as the National Old People's Welfare Committee which was subsequently to become the National Old People's Welfare Council (in both cases an offshoot of the National Council of Social Service). In 1970 it broke away from that council to become an independent organisation and adopted the new cover-name of Age Concern. The National Old People's Welfare Council in the twenty-four years of its life was responsible for the setting up of over 1000 Old People's Welfare Committees throughout England (Roberts, 1969). Each of these acted as a focus where various people concerned in providing voluntary help for the aged in an area could get together. Their membership thus included organisers of old people's clubs, visiting services, churches, other voluntary organisations such as the Red Cross and WRVS and some representation of the statutory social services and of the hospital geriatric service. These local committees have been able to stimulate the development of visiting services, luncheon clubs, old people's clubs, day centres, the organisation of group holidays, good neighbour services, chiropody services, meals-on-wheels and a host of other special services. They have acted as pioneering bodies, both in providing new services and in exploring the need for volunteers to have some form of training. The national organisation, Age Concern, has acted as a resource body to all the local committees and at the same time, plays a national role in striving for improvements in the quality of life of old people by commissioning research, lobbying Members of Parliament, producing national publications and organising seminars, conferences, etc.

Another important voluntary organisation is the Pre-retirement Association. This also has a national headquarters and a network of local committees throughout the country. Their commitment is the establishment of pre-retirement training courses. The basic pattern is that employers should allow their employees to attend such courses one day a week, usually for eight to ten weeks, and usually five to ten years before they are due to retire. The implications of retirement are considered from the financial, social, morale, housing, health and many other points of view. The pre-retirement movement is now gathering impetus, although it still only involves a very small proportion of potential old age pensioners and its work awaits evaluation.

TEACHING AND GERIATRICS

New medical specialties are rather like new religious sects in the enthusiastic missionary zeal with which they tend to preach their gospel. Geriatric medicine has been no exception and from the earliest times its practitioners have lost no opportunity to inculcate the special medical problems of old people and the need for a positive approach to their care. Perhaps one of the earliest statements was Marjorie Warren's paper in the *Lancet* of 1943 entitled *A Case for Treating Chronic Sick in Blocks in a General Hospital.'*

The specialty struggled to achieve its identity throughout the 1940s and 1950s in the face of many sceptical physicians who felt that they were doing all that was needed towards the medical care of old people. The justification for the existence of a separate specialty is the fact that the total care of old people cannot be contained within the normal system by which internal medicine is practised: indeed it has more in common with the system of care practised by the general practitioner. As will be apparent from the descriptions above of a geriatric service, the geriatrician, whilst first and foremost a clinician, has as his special interests physical rehabilitation, the management of the day hospital, the management of long-term care, the encouragement of a preventive service and the overall development of a total area medical service for elderly people.

Teaching has involved particularly student nurses, student health visitors, student district nurses, students of speech therapy, physiotherapy, occupational therapy, social workers and more recently those taking courses for wardens of sheltered housing and managers of residential homes (Brocklehurst, 1974). There is now a Post-basic Certificate in Geriatric Nursing with a nationally recognised curriculum and examination (Board of Clinical Nursing Studies 1972.) This is a six-month course for registered or enrolled nurses and it will undoubtedly do much to raise the standard of geriatric nursing.

Geriatrics has always been an important subject in postgraduate medical courses reflecting the inadequacy which many general practitioners have felt in handling the increasing numbers of old people on their practice lists. Perhaps the most important development, however, has been the achievement of academic status by the specialty and the setting up of university chairs of which there are now eight in the country, and more to come. This has marked the recognition of the need for medical undergraduates to receive teaching in geriatric medicine. It cannot but improve the understanding of the specialty and in the long-term raise the quality of its practice.

The training of a specialist in geriatric medicine is similar to that of other medical and surgical specialists. It involves three or four years' training in general medicine following registration (including the obtaining of the Diploma of MRCP in a highly competitive examination). Having completed this successfully, the doctor may then proceed to two to four years of specialist training and only at the end of that time may he compete for consultant appointments in the National Health Service. It is exceptional, therefore, for consultants to be appointed under the age of 30 and, indeed, they are usually several years older than this.

The setting up of the academic units has also acted as a stimulus for research both into aspects of geriatric medicine and in the various branches of gerontology.

The British Geriatrics Society, which was founded in 1948 as the Society for Medical Care of the Elderly, is the chief professional group involved in the struggle for recognition of the specialty and for the deployment of more adequate resources. It has issued memoranda based on detailed discussion and research on many aspects of geriatric care and many of these have formed the basis of advisory memoranda subsequently issued by the Ministry of Health. The British Geriatrics Society at present has a membership of 650, all of whom are medical practitioners with a major interest or involvement in care for old people. It has suggested standards for nurse staffing, medical staffing, staffing by therapists, problems of recruitment, vocational training, teaching, use of residential accommodation, geriatric day hospitals, etc.

THE PRESENT STATUS OF GERIATRICS

Despite its enormous development in the last quarter century from four or five consultants in 1948 to nearly 300 at the time of writing, there is no doubt that geriatrics still remains one of the less popular specialties and recruitment at the present time is a matter for grave concern. This reflects of course the present shortage of medical graduates in Great Britain and the fact that over one-quarter of doctors practising in the United Kingdom are immigrants who were not trained at British medical schools and who, in the great majority of cases, were trained either in India or Pakistan. During a period of ten months between 1970 and 1972, twenty-four consultant appointments in geriatric medicine were advertised, only fourteen of these were filled and in seven cases with an overseas graduate. This compares with an overall number of 306 posts filled throughout all specialties during that period of time in which sixty-four (21%) were overseas graduates. This recruitment of 50% of consultants from non-British graduates compares with other specialties as follows:

Opthalmology	45%
Radiology	30%
Psychiatry and Anaesthetics	25%
General Medicine	17%
General Surgery	11%

In fact in 1975 the entire British National Health Service faces a staffing crisis of unprecedented proportions. There are approximately 1000 unfilled consultant appointments throughout the country. The life earnings in general practice are, at the present time, higher than in specialist practice, the successful outcome of a government-sponsored scheme to improve recruitment into general practice. It has, however, reflected particularly adversely on the less popular hospital specialties. During the next few years the output of doctors from the medical schools will rise quite considerably and, therefore, some improvement is to be expected.

All specialists within the British National Health Service are paid a salary based on the number of sessions they work each week. A whole-time appointment is equivalent to eleven sessions, but consultants may opt for a maximum part-time appointment of nine sessions. The consultant carrying out the nine sessions is assumed to undertake the same amount of work as one who carries out eleven sessions, but the former may also engage in private practice, which is forbidden to the latter. Salary scales are also augmented by distinction awards for about one-third of hospital specialists. These are awarded in secret and generally geriatrics has not done as well as other specialties, although there is now a trend towards improvement.

PROBLEMS THAT REMAIN

The most obvious remaining problem in the development of geriatric services in Great Britain is that of undercapitalisation. A tense equilibrium exists between the increasing numbers of dependent old people on the one hand and the resources that may be deployed for their assistance on the other hand. This equilibrium is upset from time to time, either by peaks of excessive frustration and anger at individual examples of neglect or at the inadequacy of the service and, on the other hand, by political decisions as to the deployment of resources in the National Health Service and indeed within all public services. This is affected by political stop-go mechanisms, when all capital expansion is frozen because of increasing phases of difficulty in the national economy. This has last happened in 1974.

Examples of the former were the publication of the book *Sans Everything* by an organisation called AEGIS headed by Mrs Barbara Robb (1967). This gave documented stories of individual items of neglect and indeed of cruelty, mainly within the large mental hospitals, but also involving geriatric patients. As a result of this type of pressure a larger proportion of Health Service resources has moved towards geriatrics in the early 1970s than at any other time in the Health Service and a number of new units were completed during this time.

Geriatric care is relatively cheap compared to other types of medical care, but because of the low status of the specialty within individual hospital groups, individual consultants have often had great difficulty in achieving adequate priorities for their schemes of development. Indeed, in a number of major hospitals, whole new ward blocks, which have been specially designed and built for geriatric patients, have had their use diverted, once they were completed, for medicine and surgery.

One interesting and important outcome arising from *Sans Everything* and other press reports, was the setting up of the Hospital Advisory Service by the Department of Health and Social Security. This is an independent advisory organisation staffed by doctors, nurses, therapists and administrators. It was set up in 1970 and since then has visited most of the geriatric and psychiatric hospitals in the country and issued annual reports on its findings.

In this report for 1971 the Director of the Hospital Advisory Service, Dr A A Baker, said,

> 'I am placing the Geriatric Hospital Service in the forefront of my report, as in my opinion, these services now require the greatest concentration of effort and resources. The geriatric services have probably occupied a "Cinderella" position ever since they began to

emerge as a separate specialty. It is surprising, however, that in view of the widespread recognition of the increasing problem caused by our elderly population, so little priority is being given to developing this branch of medicine. Even in planning for future general hospitals it is common to find that far too few beds are being allocated to a geriatric service and in existing hospitals it is almost always the case that the geriatrician is given the worst accommodation and the rejects from other specialties'.

The Director then goes on to refer to geriatric hospitals where patients have to be carried up and down stairs in chairs and where the toilet doors are not wide enough to take a wheelchair.

> 'A mile or two away, on a fine open site, there is a modern building for the physicians, surgeons and others, with every modern facility, adequate car parking and full ancillary services. Is it surprising that there is difficulty in recruiting another geriatrician and that beds are blocked?'

The report for 1972 details the procedure by which the Director of the Service had letters sent to a number of recently discharged patients before a visit to an individual hospital. He was impressed by the seriousness of the replies, by the fact that many correspondents commented that never before had they been asked to give their opinion on a public service and that the majority of letters were full of praise for the care and kindness they received. As far as complaints were concerned the report goes on:

> The commonest complaints refer to the effects of custodial care and regimentation. For example:
>
> "I quickly became very bored with doing nothing and would have liked some activity to help pass the time."
>
> "They woke me with a bowl of water at 5.0 am but I did not get a cup of tea until 7.30 am. The radio was turned on at 8.0 am and left on and we had to bear it. Luckily it was turned off for doctors' visits."
>
> "The thing that did bore me was that we had to sit in the day room for seven or eight hours and I got very depressed."
>
> "The patients should be allowed to rest, when they are old, on their beds in the afternoon. I got very tired sitting about all day as it is a very long day."
>
> "Our personal clothing was all taken from us and we had to wear hospital dressing gowns and nightdresses. There seemed to be a

shortage of these and as I was not incontinent, I had to wear mine for three weeks."

"We were treated like children. We all had to wear bibs at mealtimes whether we were untidy or not."

"They will not let me have my own clothing. My daughter would do the washing, but they will not let me have it."

"We patients had to sit in the same chair all day and every day." '

In discussing attitudes of colleagues towards geriatric medicine, the Director goes on to say,

'Unfortunately hostility to geriatrics and to geriatric staff can be found at all levels in the hospital service and I am sorry to say that prejudice and lack of understanding can occur amongst the most eminent in a Teaching Hospital as well as in the most isolated rural group. For example, a Professor of a well-known Teaching Hospital was heard to say that "medical students should not be contaminated by contact with geriatric patients." At another hospital, the senior physician said, "geriatricians are undesirable". These attitudes to professional colleagues and their patients are a serious reflection on a profession usually noted for its concern for the sick, handicapped and under-privileged. In the past it may have appeared that nothing could be done about old people with long-term handicap, but young and enthusiastic geriatricians have shown that something can be done.'

Perhaps the most important single problem that remains is the need for hospital buildings which are designed especially for the care of old people. Probably the majority of buildings still occupied by old people were put up in the 19th Century.

New developments at the present time include an increasing interest in the field of psycho-geriatrics, a liaison in relation to the care of patients with fracture of the femur, the emergence of young chronic sick units as separate parts of the hospital service and no longer necessarily in the charge of the geriatrician and an awakening interest in the care of the dying.

Psycho-geriatrics

Perhaps the most serious single problem for the future is going to be the management of the increasing number of patients suffering from senile dementia. The cause of this chronically debilitating disease is as yet unknown and there is no specific treatment. The demented old person may for a period of two or three years or longer be quite unable to look after herself, and if living with her family, may provoke almost intolerable stress. The stress caused in families has been alluded to in many geriatric surveys beginning with that of Sheldon (1947) who reported some form of stress generated by old people in private households in 7% of people aged 65 and over he investigated.

At one time most of these old people were admitted directly to the large mental hospitals, but it has become the accepted policy of the last few years that wherever possible these large isolated mental hospitals should be run down and psychiatric departments should be developed within general hospitals. This has exacerbated the problem of the confused old person and various solutions have been experimented with. The whole subject is well-reviewed in *The Elderly Mind* (1972).

A pattern of psycho-geriatric care has now been accepted by the Department of Health which has laid down guidelines including bed norms for this purpose. Guidance was offered in 1970 on the setting-up of psycho-geriatric assessment units (HMSO 70/11). It was suggested that a unit of this kind should be set up in each proposed district general hospital; that it should be of between ten and twenty beds for a population of 250 000 people and that the maximum length of stay should be four weeks. The unit was to be managed with the closest cooperation between the geriatric physician and the psychiatrist, but should remain the clinical responsibility of one of these consultants.

Subsequent guidance (HMSO 72/71) considered the question of long-stay care for confused old people. They were divided into three groups. First, those who had grown old in hospitals for the mentally ill—often after having been there for many years. This was thought to be a diminishing problem and that the most humane method of dealing with it was to leave most of these aging people in the surroundings that were familiar to them. The second group were elderly patients with functional mental illness, including the small minority needing longer-stay care. They should be contained within the general provision of psychiatric beds and day places.

The third group were those suffering from dementia, including confusional disorders and these were divided again into three groups; (*a*) those with mild dementia, not suffering from significant physical disease (*b*) those with more severe dementia, not suffering from significant physical disease and (*c*) those with dementia, whether mild or severe, who were also suffering from significant physical disease.

In general it was felt that the first group (*a*) with appropriate care and support, could be looked after either at home or in local authority residential homes. The third group (*c*) were regarded as being properly the responsibility of the geriatric department to be looked after within the bed provision for geriatrics. The second group were regarded as falling neither within the psychiatric nor the geriatric hospital commitment and for this group of patients a new type of psycho-geriatric long-stay care was proposed providing two and a half to three beds and one to two day places per 1000 persons aged 65 and over.

Following these recommendations there has been a long discussion and the gradual emergence of a pattern of psycho-geriatric care in parallel with geriatric care on the one hand and psychiatric care on the other.

CONCLUSION

This account of the development of medical services for old people in Great Britain has emphasised the problems that have beset this process and the way in which some have been overcome. Despite the shortcomings that still remain, however, there is no doubt that the progress that has been made in the quarter century since the setting up of the National Health Service has been very real and a high standard of medical care is available to most old people at no immediate cost to themselves, whenever they require it. The service is humane and medically effective and is achieved in Great Britain with a proportion of institutionalised places (beds in old people's homes and in geriatric hospitals), which is less than that in most other countries. On the whole, the service is well-administered and patients are well-investigated before long-term hospital care is accepted as a necessity. Every attempt is made to support people in their own homes and this is successful to a remarkable extent.

What now remains to be done is to afford greater dignity and privacy to the old people using these services. More emphasis is required on the quality of life in long-stay wards and old people's homes and an additional drive is needed to diminish the length of time old people must wait before they receive appropriate care. More emphasis must be placed on the ascertainment of unreported illness and in preventive health generally, in and before old age. A more positive attitude is required towards the worth of old people and the importance of providing for their care by all health service professionals. And finally, there is still need for diversion of a larger proportion of resources in their direction.

References

Anderson, W. F. and Cowan, N. R. (1955). A consultative Health Centre for older people. *Lancet,* **ii,** 239-40

Andrews, C. T. (1971). Early days in rural England. *Modern Geriatrics,* **1,** 117-121

Bright, R. (1972). *Music in Geriatric Care* (London: Angus and Robertson)
Brocklehurst, J. C. and Shergold, M. (1969). Old people leaving hospital. *Gerontol Clin.*, **ii,** 115-26
Brocklehurst, J. C. (1970). *The Geriatric Day Hospital* (King Edwards Hospital Fund for London)
Brocklehurst, J. C. (1974). *Textbook of Geriatric Medicine and Gerontology* (Edinburgh and London: Churchill Livingstone)
Brocklehurst, J. C. (1974). Educational opportunities in geriatrics. *Age and Aging,* **3,** 3-11
The Board of Clinical Nursing Studies (1972). Outline curriculum in geriatric nursing for state registered and state enrolled nurses, **Course No. 296**
Buckingham County Council (1973). Social Services Department. *A Study of Residents Admitted to Buckingham County Welfare Homes*
Davies, L., Hastrop, K. and Bender, A. E. (1974). Meals on wheels. *Modern Geriatrics,* **4,** 468-474
Department of Health and Social Security (1970). *Psychogeriatric Assessment Units,* 70 (11) (London: HMSO)
Department of Health and Social Security (1972). *Services for Mental Illness Related to Old Age,* 72 (71). (London: HMSO)
Eckstein, H. and Harvard, U. P. (1958). *The English Health Service* (Cambridge, Mass., British Health Care and Technology)
The Elderly Mind (1972). (British Hospital Journal, Hospital International, London)
Exton-Smith, A. N. and Stanton, B. R. (1972). *Nutrition of Housebound Old People* (King Edward's Hospital Fund for London)
Farndale, W. J. (1961). *The Day Hospital Movement in Great Britain* (Oxford: Pergamon Press)
Flowers, J. and Parry, Noel C. A., (1974). *Old Age in Hertfordshire* (A Report for the Hertfordshire Social Services Department)
General Medical Services (1973). *Report of a Joint Working Party* (London: HMSO)
Harris, A. I. (1971). *Handicapped and Impaired in Great Britain* (London: HMSO)
Halliburton, P. M. and Wright, W. B. (1973). Variations in standard of hospital geriatric care. *Lancet,* **i,** 1300-02.
Hodgkinson, Ruth G. (1967). *The Origins of the National Health Service.* The medical services of the new poor law, 1834-1871 (London: Wellcome Historical Medical Library)
Lowther, C. P., Macleod, R. D. M. and Williamson, J. (1970). Evaluation of early diagnostic services for the elderly. *Brit. Med. J.,* 275-7

Poulden, Sylvia M. (1971). Art in the geriatric ward. *Brit. Hosp. J. & Social Services Review,* 29th May

Prinsley, D. N. (1971). Effects of industrial action by the ambulance service on day hospital patients. *Brit. Med. J.,* **ii,** 170-1

Robb, Barbara. (1967). *Sans Everything* (London: Thos. Nelson)

Roberts, Nesta (1970). *Our Future Selves* (London: George Allen and Unwin Ltd.)

Roth, M., Kay, D. W. K., and Beamish, P. (1964). Old age mental disorders in Newcastle Upon Tyne. *Brit. J. Psychiatry,* **110,** 146-58

Shanus, R. (1968). *Old People in Three Industrial Societies* (London: Routledge and Kegan Paul)

Sheldon, J. H. (1948). *The Social Medicine of Old Age* (London: The Nuffield Foundation)

Speed, M. G. (1971). *The Year Book of Social Policy in Britain* (London: Routledge and Kegan Paul)

Stanton, B. R. (1971). *Meals for the Elderly* (King Edward's Hospital Fund for London)

Townsend, P. (1964). *The Last Refuge* (London: Routledge and Kegan Paul)

Townsend, P. and Wedderburn, D. (1965). *The Aged in the Welfare State. Papers in Social Administration* (London: Bell)

Warren, M. W. (1943). A case for treating chronic sick in blocks in a general hospital. *Brit. Med. J.,* 822-3

Warren, M. W. (1949). The role of a geriatric unit in a general hospital. *Ulster Med. J.,* 3-12

Williams, E. I., Bennett, F. M., Nixon, J. V., Nicholson, R. M. and Gabert, J. (1972). Sociomedical study of patients over 75 in general medical practice. *Brit. Med. J.,* **ii,** 445-8

Williamson, J., Stokoe, I. H., Gray, S., Fisher, M., Smith, A., McGhee, A. and Stephenson, E. (1964). Old people at home: their unreported needs. *Lancet,* **i,** 1117-20

Williamson, J., Lowther, C. P. and Grey, S. (1966). The use of health visitors in preventive geriatrics. *Gerontol. Clin.,* **8,** 362-9

CHAPTER THREE

The Netherlands

R J van Zonneveld

INTRODUCTION

The Netherlands belong to those industrialised countries of Europe, North America and Australia which have a relatively high percentage of people 65 years of age and over (the so-called 'old people'). In all these 'western' countries this percentage is ten or more. Besides being industrialised these countries are characterised by rapid urbanisation, increased bureaucracy, automatisation and often *miniaturisation* of working activities. These aspects of technological development, changes in ethics and the greater emphasis on youth together with an increase in the percentage of 'old people' have led in all western countries to the so-called 'problem of the aged'. Whether there really exists such a problem, or whether it is as great a problem as some authors try to make us believe needs to be questioned. If there is such a real problem, it has arisen in the present century when society has focused its interest on the younger section of the population.

In the Netherlands as in other industrially developed countries the birthrate has been decreasing continuously during the last four or five decades—with brief exceptions—so that inevitably the percentage of old people has increased.

SOME DEMOGRAPHIC DATA

The Netherlands is a small country with a surface area of about 26854 km^2. The proximity of the North Sea through which the gulf stream passes, gives Holland (the name often given to the Netherlands—in fact it is a *pars pro toto;* the Netherlands consist of eleven provinces, two of which are named South and North Holland) a moderate climate with mild, wet winters and in general cool wet summers. The western part of the country—which is also the most densely populated part—is also subject to strong winds. Colds, influenza and influenza-like types of respiratory diseases, asthma, bronchitis and pneumonia are therefore prevalent among the aged. The saying in the past that pneumonia was the old man's friend, applied in the Netherlands. The prevailing west wind causes much hindrance, particularly to old pedestrians and cyclists. On the other hand, by far the greater part of the country is flat, which reduces the strain on the heart muscle.

The population (in 1974) is 13.5 million, of which 10.4% is 65 years and over (i.e. 1.4 million). This percentage is smaller than in Northern, Central and Western Europe. In fact from this point of view the Netherlands have the youngest population; in Belgium 13.6% of the population is 65 and over; in the Federal Republic of Germany 13.5%; in France 13.0%; in Italy 10.9%; in Great Britain 13.2% and in Denmark 13.6% (all figures for 1972). The Democractic Republic of Germany has the highest percentage; in 1974, of a population of 17.6 million, 3 335 000 were pensioners—mostly over 60 (women) or over 65 (men). This relatively low percentage of old people in Holland has been caused by the high birthrate during past years in this country (in 1958 it was still 21.2/1000 , in 1969 it was 19.2/1000 and in 1973 it was 14.6/1000) and by relatively very little emigration since 1955. During the first decade after World War II some considerable emigration took place.

The percentage of old people began to increase in the 1930s: in 1899 the percentage was 6.0, whilst in 1930 it was 6.2; in 1960 it was 10.0 and in 1971 it was 10.2. According to calculations by the Netherlands' Central Bureau of Statistics the percentage in the future will further increase to 11.1 or 11.2 in 1980 and 11.7-12.1 in the year 2000, but will then still be less than the present figures in several surrounding countries.

While the aging of the population as a whole will therefore continue in a moderate way, the aging within the group aged 65 years and older will be much more rapid (Table 3.1).

Those aged over 80 and particularly those over 85 years will increase most rapidly—particularly women. Of the old people aged 80-85 years 58.5% (1973) are female. Of those aged 95 and over 60.2% are female. Thus the group consisting of the oldest women is increasing most rapidly. From many surveys (e.g. van Zonneveld, 1961 a) it is known that many more old women than old men are ill or disabled. Therefore, as

Table 3.1 Aging within the group of old people (Figures from the Netherlands' Central Bureau of Statistics)

Year	*65-69*	*70-74*	*75-79*	*80 a.o.*	*Total*
1951	38.8	29.6	18.5	13.1	100
1961	37.4	28.2	19.0	15.4	100
1971	36.1	27.6	19.3	17.0	100

elsewhere, geriatrics is particularly concerned with the oldest age-groups of women.

This group also consists mostly of single persons (widows, divorcees, spinsters) who therefore need more help in cases of physical and/or mental disease or disability. Fortunately the percentage of married couples of 65 and over is slowly increasing. The percentage of married old men is also increasing, while that of married old women is rising more slowly (Table 3.2).

Table 3.2 Married old people in 1899, 1947 and 1971

Year	*men %*	*women %*	*total %*	*% difference between men and women*
1899	56.3	34.2	44.2	22.1
1947	62.6	42.6	52.1	20.0
1971	72.2	43.8	55.3	28.4

In the age-group of 80 years and over there are twice as many married old men as married old women. This can be explained by the fact that there are many men of 65 and over married to women younger than 65. Men also remain married longer because the average life expectancy of women is longer. Moreover, more men remarry at higher ages than women (de Mast *et al.*, 1972).

Life expectancy for the married is higher than for the single. For the unmarried and widowed it is higher than for the divorced. In the period 1961-1965 life expectancy for people at 65 years of age is shown in Table 3.3. According to more recent data (1972) life expectancy at birth is 70.8

Table 3.3 Life expectancy at age 65 (in years) (1961-1965)

	Men	*Women*
Married	14.3	16.1
Single	13.2	15.6
Divorced	11.2	15.4

years for men and 76.0 for women; at the age of 65 expectancy is 13.4 and 16.6 years respectively.

Attention has been directed to these few demographic data, because the figures have direct relevance to the types and extent of care for the aged.

Mortality

Since seven out of each ten persons in the Netherlands die after the age of 65, it is self-evident that the three major causes of death for the total population are also the most important causes of death in old people. In order of importance they are (1968): cardiovascular diseases (22% of all deaths up to 65 years, 36% of all deaths from 65 years), malignant neoplasms (31% and 22% respectively) and diseases of nervous system and senses, i.e. mostly cerebrovascular diseases (7% and 16% respectively). The fourth important cause of death in old people is disease of the respiratory tract (nearly 7%) and the fifth is accidents, intoxications and violence (4%). In absolute numbers these data mean that in 1972 42 700 old people died because of diseases of the circulatory organs (of these about 12 000 of cerebrovascular disorders), 17 700 of malignant growths, 6300 of respiratory diseases and 2900 because of accidents, intoxications and violence. The cause of death described according to 'The International Statistical Classification of Diseases, Injuries and Causes of Death' as old-age symptoms and badly described conditions was in 1972 given as 1068 persons younger than 65 and 3100 persons older than 65.

In old age itself some diseases are becoming gradually more important causes of death, other less (Table 3.4). In people from 65-69 years of age,

Table 3.4 % of total number of deaths in different age groups in 1967

	65-69	*80-84*	*85+*
Cerebrovascular	11.4	18.9	17.2
Cardiovascular	33.7	37.5	39.6
Malignant tumours	32.5	18.4	13.5

the five main causes of death are in order of importance (1967): cardiovascular diseases (33.7%), malignant neoplasms (32.5%), diseases of the nervous system and sense (11.4%), diseases of respiratory system (5.1%) and accidents (3.6%). In people of 85 and over the order is: cardiovascular diseases (39.6%), cerebrovascular diseases (17.2%), malignant growths (13.5%), respiratory diseases (6.8%) and old age etc. (6.0%).

According to the Dutch notification system *one* cause of death must be indicated as the most important cause; the cause 'old age, etc.' is not easily accepted by the Central Bureau of Statistics. Therefore the data given above only present a rough picture: in old people often several diseases may present simultaneously and doctors are encouraged to notify a specific cause rather than to state that they do not know the real cause. Thus, the approximate number of 2000 old persons having died of old age symptoms and badly described conditions, is relatively low; in countries where there is less emphasis on notifying specific causes, the category last mentioned (old age etc.) is much more common, e.g. in Portugal, for the age-group of 80 and over in 35-40% of the cases. On calculations made by the Netherlands' Central Bureau of Statistics it is expected that in 1980 about 22 300 men of 65 and over and 18 200 women of 65 and over will die of cardiovascular diseases and that 13 500 old men and 9000 old women will die of cancer.

From the above data it is seen that care of old people with cardiovascular disease becomes somewhat more important as they reach very high ages. This is even more the case for cerebrovascular diseases but less so for malignant neoplasms. In fact when one looks especially at patients in nursing-homes, a great number of them are hemiplegics. The nursing-home has thus in the Netherlands become the institution where, generally speaking, the most adequate treatment is given to victims of stroke.

Morbidity

Comparatively little is known about diseases and disability among the aged. A nation-wide survey on the health of 3149 old people examined by 374 (their own) general practitioners, performed in 1955-1957 (van Zonneveld, 1961 b) shed some light on this matter, as do some local investigations.

The following tables derived from the first-mentioned survey give data respectively on the frequency, by sex and five-year age-groups on the kind of principal affection for which the old people* received their last medical treatment (Table 3.5), for which a physician was regularly consulted (Table 3.6), for which a specialist was consulted after the age of 65, (Table 3.7) and for which hospitalisation occurred after the age of 65 (Table 3.8).

Table 3.5 shows that cardiovascular and renal disease took first place (19-33%) with a significantly higher percentage for women than men in

*Random samples in each sex and age-group of the total population of 65 and over, with the exception of those ± 2% who were treated in hospitals or nursing-homes by special doctors

all age groups with the exception of the group of 80-84 years. The group of 'other diseases' follows (18-28%) with almost identical percentages for both sexes. The group of diseases of the respiratory system (excluding neoplasms and tuberculosis) is very important (12-24%), with the men leading significantly in all age-groups but one. The oldest group of men and the oldest group of women differ inversely. About one in thirty women reported that the last treatment was primarily for diabetes, an appreciable proportion.

Table 3.6 shows the group of principal diseases for which a physician was regularly consulted. Almost half of the men and of the women who saw a doctor regularly did so for cardiovascular and renal diseases. On this point there was no important difference between the sexes. Among the remaining groups of diseases for which a doctor was consulted regularly there was none especially remarkable for great frequency. 'Rheumatic' affections took second place among women, respiratory affections were second among men and third for women.

The data in Table 3.7 are more or less in agreement with those shown in Table 3.6. More women than men consulted a specialist after the age of 65, although the difference is less marked than might have been expected and not significant. The specialist was again most often consulted for disorders in the category of cardiovascular and renal diseases, though the group of 'other diseases' was here much more important than in the preceding case. This latter group, however, usually includes the consulting of an ophthalmologist for eyeglasses. Men consulted a specialist for a prostate disorder in 4, 8, 13, 18 and 27% in the successive age-groups.

Finally, Table 3.8 indicates the principal reasons for being admitted into a hospital after the age of 65; 16-45% of the men and 21-40% of the women in the sample were admitted to hospital one or more times. Age is again an important factor. Those who had only recently reached 65 had had much less chance of hospitalisation than those who had long since passed this age. Not only may the younger aged have had less illness requiring hospitalisation, but they may also have had more possibility of being nursed elsewhere than in a hospital. Such factors are implied in the results shown in Table 3.8.

The visits of referral to a specialist are of course different from those to a general practitioner. Some disorders rate more frequently, such as prostate conditions, while others become relatively less important, i.e. not only cardiovascular and renal diseases but also respiratory disorders. Thus while 65 men reported their last visit to the doctor to have been primarily for prostate trouble, only 28 regularly consulted a physician for this condition. However, after the age of 65, a specialist was

Table 3.5 Kind of principal affection for which last medical treatment was received; by sex and age-groups; percentages

Age	Cardio-vascular and renal diseases	Malignant neoplasms	Cerebral and mental diseases (suicide), apoplexy	Gastro-intestinal diseases	Diseases of the respiratory system	Tuber-culosis	Infective diseases	Prostate complaints	Rheuma-tism	Diabetes (only)	Other diseases	Total %	Total Abs
Men													
65–69	20.7	1.2	1.5	10.7	21.6	0.9	3.7	2.1	7.0	2.4	28.2	100	328
70–74	21.7	1.3	3.4	10.4	21.1	1.3	2.9	3.4	7.0	2.1	25.4	100	383
75–79	25.4	1.6	3.4	10.9	21.7	–	4.1	4.7	8.0	1.3	18.9	100	387
80–84	29.4	1.8	1.1	5.1	24.2	0.4	4.0	5.8	4.0	4.7	19.5	100	277
85+	19.1	4.6	3.1	8.4	19.8	–	3.8	8.4	3.8	0.8	28.2	100	131
Total	23.9	1.7	2.5	9.4	21.8	0.6	3.7	4.3	6.4	2.3	23.4	100	1506
Women													
65–69	26.5	3.9	3.9	11.4	12.3	0.3	1.8	–	11.4	3.0	25.5	100	333
70–74	31.7	3.4	3.7	7.9	13.1	0.8	2.1	–	10.5	3.7	23.1	100	382
75–79	33.4	2.4	3.2	11.2	12.3	–	2.1	–	8.6	4.0	22.8	100	374
80–84	28.6	2.3	5.6	10.5	12.8	0.8	2.3	–	10.2	2.6	24.3	100	266
85+	29.4	3.3	5.3	7.3	24.0	–	4.0	–	4.7	4.0	18.0	100	150
Total	30.0	3.1	4.1	9.9	13.8	0.4	2.3	–	9.6	3.5	23.3	100	1505

Table 3.6 Groups of principal diseases for which a physician was regularly consulted; by sex and age-groups; percentages

Ages	No regular consult-ations	Regular consultation on:										Total	
		Cardio-vascular and renal diseases	Malignant neoplasms	Cerebral and mental diseases (suicide), apoplexy	Gastro-intestinal diseases	Diseases of the respiratory system	Infective diseases	Prostate complaints	Rheuma-tism	Diabetes (only)	Other diseases	%	Abs
Men													
65-69	64.6	15.1	0.9	2.0	4.3	3.4	–	0.9	2.3	1.4	5.1	100	351
70-74	68.5	14.3	0.5	2.0	2.5	4.4	0.5	1.2	1.7	1.0	3.4	100	406
75-79	62.0	18.0	0.5	3.2	1.9	5.4	0.5	1.7	1.2	3.9	3.9	100	411
80-84	57.9	20.3	0.7	0.7	1.7	4.7	0.3	3.1	1.4	4.1	4.1	100	295
85+	59.2	13.1	2.9	0.7	2.2	7.3	–	2.9	2.2	7.3	7.3	100	137
Total	63.2	16.4	0.8	2.1	2.6	4.8	0.3	1.8	1.8	4.4	4.4	100	1600
Women													
65-69	50.9	19.8	3.2	2.9	5.7	1.1	0.3	–	6.6	3.2	6.3	100	348
70-74	42.4	27.4	2.0	2.3	2.0	2.0	3.8	–	6.4	3.1	10.3	100	391
75-79	42.4	27.0	1.3	1.0	4.7	4.5	–	–	5.2	3.7	10.2	100	382
80-84	43.1	23.6	1.8	4.4	3.0	3.7	0.4	–	6.3	4.1	9.6	100	271
85+	47.3	23.7	2.6	6.6	2.0	5.3	–	–	4.6	2.6	5.3	100	152
Total	45.0	24.5	2.1	2.9	3.7	3.5	0.2	–	6.0	3.4	8.7	100	1544

Table 3.7 Groups of principal diseases for which a specialist was consulted after the age of 65 years; by sex and age-groups; percentages

Ages	No consultations	Consultation of a specialist after the 65th year of age because of: Cardio-vascular and renal diseases	Malignant neoplasms	Cerebral and mental diseases (suicide), apoplexy	Gastro-intestinal diseases	Diseases of the respiratory system	Infective diseases	Prostate complaints	Rheumatism	Diabetes (only)	Other diseases	Total %	Total Abs
Men													
65-69	62.7	8.3	1.1	1.7	4.8	2.8	0.6	1.7	2.6	0.6	13.1	100	351
70-74	47.6	10.8	1.7	2.7	8.6	2.7	0.5	4.2	3.4	1.5	16.3	100	406
75-79	42.7	8.3	2.4	2.4	7.1	4.9	0.2	7.6	3.2	1.2	20.0	100	409
80-84	44.0	7.1	2.0	1.0	7.8	3.7	0.7	10.2	2.7	3.1	17.7	100	294
85+	44.2	2.2	4.3	0.7	5.1	2.2	–	15.2	2.2	1.4	22.5	100	138
Total	48.8	8.2	2.1	1.9	6.9	3.4	0.4	6.6	2.9	1.5	17.3	100	1598
Women													
65-69	54.2	7.5	3.5	2.0	6.9	1.4	0.3	–	4.9	2.6	16.7	100	347
70-74	39.8	11.5	3.6	2.0	7.7	2.3	0.8	–	5.9	3.6	22.8	100	391
75-79	37.4	11.6	3.2	0.5	13.2	2.4	0.8	–	2.4	3.2	25.3	100	380
80-84	46.6	7.4	3.7	0.4	5.9	2.2	–	–	3.7	2.6	27.5	100	269
85+	50.0	4.6	2.0	2.6	7.9	1.3	–	–	–	2.0	29.6	100	152
Total	44.7	9.2	3.3	1.4	8.6	2.0	0.5	–	3.8	2.9	23.6	100	1539

Table 3.8 Groups of principal diseases for which hospitalisation occurred after the age of 65; by sex and age-groups; percentages

		Admission into a hospital after 65th year of age because of										Total	
Ages	*No hospital-isation*	*Cardio-vascular and renal diseases*	*Malignant neoplasms*	*Cerebral and mental diseases (suicide), apoplexy*	*Gastro-intestinal diseases*	*Diseases of the respiratory system*	*Infective diseases*	*Prostate complaints*	*Rheuma-tism*	*Diabetes (only)*	*Other diseases*	*%*	*Abs*
Men													
65-69	83.9	3.7	0.9	0.9	2.0	1.1	0.3	1.4	0.6	0.9	4.3	100	351
70-74	70.8	5.2	1.5	1.2	5.4	2.5	0.7	3.4	0.7	0.5	8.1	100	407
75-79	63.0	4.1	2.0	1.0	6.1	2.4	0.2	7.1	0.7	0.7	12.7	100	410
80-84	55.5	3.7	1.0	0.7	7.5	1.4	0.7	12.2	0.3	1.4	15.6	100	295
85+	58.0	1.4	2.2	0.7	8.0	2.2	–	13.8	0.7	1.4	11.6	100	138
Total	68.0	4.0	1.4	0.9	5.4	1.9	0.4	6.4	0.6	0.9	10.1	100	1601
Women													
65-69	79.5	3.2	2.0	0.9	4.3	0.6	0.3	–	1.1	0.6	7.5	100	348
70-74	66.6	4.8	3.6	1.5	4.8	2.6	0.5	–	1.3	1.8	12.5	100	392
75-79	59.9	6.6	3.2	0.5	11.1	1.8	0.8	–	0.8	1.8	13.5	100	380
80-84	64.0	4.1	3.0	0.7	7.0	1.5	–	–	0.4	1.9	17.4	100	380
85+	63.1	2.6	2.0	2.0	6.6	2.0	1.3	–	–	0.7	19.7	100	152
Total	67.2	4.5	2.9	1.0	6.8	1.7	0.5	–	0.8	1.4	13.2	100	1542

seen in 105 cases and 103 were hospitalised. The figures for diabetes as the principal disease show a quite different picture: for men 35, 29, 24, and 14 cases in order of successive age-groups, and for women 52, 52, 45, and 22 cases.

Some data are available on the degree of independence of old people. In Rotterdam (population approximately 650 000 at the time) 2697 aged persons were examined on their activities of daily living in the late sixties. One or more of eleven activities of daily living (ADL) had been lost in 12% of 1212 men and 19.2% of 1485 women over the age of 65. The total number of times per sex that one of the ADL-criteria could not be met, is given in Table 3.9.

Table 3.9 ADL in old people in Rotterdam (From de Mast *et al.* (1972) by courtesy of van Loghum Slaterus)

	Men		*Women*			
	Number	*%*	*Number*	*%*	*% men**	*% women†*
Climbing stairs	103	28.5	209	31.3	8.5	14.1
Walking	65	18.0	130	19.5	5.4	8.8
Bathing, washing oneself	67	18.6	86	12.9	5.5	5.8
Clothing oneself	30	8.3	59	8.8	2.5	4.0
Reading	23	6.4	44	6.6	1.9	3.0
Stepping into bed	24	6.6	39	5.8	2.0	2.6
Combing hair	15	4.2	48	7.2	1.2	3.2
Using the WC	17	4.7	23	3.4	1.4	1.5
Going to sit down	6	1.7	11	1.7	0.5	0.7
Going to lie down	7	1.9	10	1.5	0.6	0.7
Eating	4	1.1	9	1.3	0.3	0.6
Total	361	100	668	100		

* Number of lost ADL in % of the total male group
† Number of lost ADL in % of the total female group

To give an idea of what old people thought themselves about their health and what their own family doctor's opinion was on their health status, Tables 3.10 and 3.11 are presented.

To an old person, how he feels is of very great importance. Table 3.10 indicates that the large majority of the subjects examined answered to the effect that they did feel themselves to be in good health, i.e. 78% (74-82%) of the men and 64% (59-68%) of the women. With increasing age the percentage of those who subjectively rated themselves as healthy dropped only very slightly. In almost every age-group, significantly more women than men complained about their state of health. It is possible that the generation to which these oldest individuals belong did not find it proper to complain or to admit that there was anything wrong with

Table 3.10 Subjective evaluation of health by the examinees; by sex and age-groups; percentages

Age	Men Evaluation					Women Evaluation				
	Good	Not so good	Bad	Total		Good	Not so good	Bad	Total	
				%	Abs				%	Abs
65-69	79.8	17.1	3.1	100	351	68.1	29.9	2.0	100	348
70-74	81.8	16.2	2.0	100	407	61.5	35.7	2.8	100	392
75-79	74.4	14.4	1.2	100	410	59.2	36.6	4.2	100	382
80-84	74.9	22.0	3.1	100	295	68.1	26.7	5.2	100	270
85+	75.9	21.2	2.9	100	137	66.2	29.1	4.7	100	148
Total	77.7	20.0	2.3	100	1600	64.0	32.4	3.6	100	1540

their health which might imply helplessness (see page 55). The percentage of the aged who found their own health poor was very small, i.e. 2% (1-3%) for the men and 4% (2-5%) for women. The last percentage rose somewhat in the successive age-groups. These percentages are only a little lower than in a survey on the health status and needs of 3000 old people, performed in Groningen in the fifties (van Zonneveld, 1954).

As shown in Table 3.11, the physician found the subjects' physical condition worse in almost every successive older group. In the youngest group of men, 18% made a less favourable (but 'not so good') impression; in the oldest group this figure was not less than 42%. For women these percentages were 25 and 49. In each age-group the percentage of men whose physical condition was considered good was

Table 3.11 Physical condition according to the general practitioner; by sex and age-groups; percentages

Age	Men Evaluation					Women Evaluation				
	Good	Not so good	Bad	Total		Good	Not so good	Bad	Total	
				%	Abs				%	Abs
65-69	82.0	15.7	2.3	100	350	75.2	23.9	0.9	100	347
70-74	81.3	18.0	0.7	100	406	65.0	32.4	2.6	100	392
75-79	70.4	26.2	3.4	100	408	55.1	39.1	5.8	100	379
80-84	64.1	32.5	3.4	100	295	49.8	41.7	8.5	100	271
85+	57.7	37.2	5.1	100	137	51.3	42.8	5.9	100	152
Total	73.5	23.9	2.6	100	1596	60.9	34.8	4.3	100	1541

larger than that of the women. Between 70 and 85 years, the differences are even more significant. The difference between the sexes was present for both the physician's impression and the subjects' own judgement of his health. It is therefore all the more remarkable that the men, who made a better impression and who, as reported, had fewer complaints, nevertheless have a higher death rate. There was also in general, a divergence between the subject's opinion of his own health and that of the physician. Here, needless to say, age plays an important part. Whereas the subject's judgement, particularly in the case of the women of 65-75, was less favourable than that of the physician, in the subsequent age-groups the reverse was the case. A possible explanation of this is the inability with increasing age of the individual to judge his condition objectively. This inability is perhaps connected with the euphoria which is rather frequent in very old people and a tendency to boast about their good health. In addition, many aged, as they get older, appear increasingly to adjust themselves and accept a poorer state of health as 'normal' for their age. It was also striking that the percentages of those whose physical condition was given as 'bad' (men 0.7-5%, women 0.9-9%) were so low.

Some other interesting local studies on the health of the aged have been carried out. To mention a few of the more important surveys: Fuldauer (1966) a general practitioner, examined all old people on his panel on their present situation. Tonino (1969) with the help of a team, did an extensive medical and social survey among 400 old inhabitants of Breda (a city of about 100 000 people). Much earlier van Zonneveld (1954) had already interviewed, with the help of medical students (near their graduation), 3000 old people in the city of Groningen (pop. 135 000) to assess their needs for some sort of domiciliary or institutional care. On a much more extensive scale this was done again in the city of Leiden (pop. 100 000) and municipalities in Frisia (Fennis and van Zonneveld, 1966-1970; Fennis, 1973). Oostvogel (1968) examined the people on a waiting list for an old people's home.

HISTORY

Some form of care of the aged has always existed in human society, although—as was often the case among nomads—it was sometimes quite negative. Old people who were no longer productive and useful to the group were banned or went of their own free will to a lonely place to die of starvation, cold, etc. Mostly—and this was particularly so in settled groups in an agrarian society—the old parents lived with their family until they died. This was also for many centuries true in the Netherlands.

Until the beginning of the 19th century the rural communities and the small cities consisted of social units of three or even four generations, in which the grandparents had an important responsibility in caring for and educating the children.

Generally speaking there was in Western Europe in the Middle Ages little interest in the problems of old age—there was little need for it. There were relatively few old people (perhaps only 2-3% or less of the population reached the age of 65) and those who survived, lived with their family. However, there was in the Middle Ages a beginning of care for the wounded, incapacitated and disabled who came back from the Crusades. For these certain institutions were established, so that they eventually could have a pleasant old age.

Soon after the Renaissance, because of a more positive attitude towards life, interest in old age revived (e.g. the Romans, *vide* Cicero): books appeared in several countries, giving advice on how to reach a very great age. The aged did not generally form a social problem. In the bigger cities more and more old people were not taken care of by their families. From about the 15th century in many Dutch communities so-called 'hofjes' (small courts) were built by employers, for certain of their former employees or servants, or by churches or other charitable religious organisations. Such 'hofjes' consisted of one or more rows of small dwellings, often grouped around a courtyard. In these small houses old people could live free or for a very low rent. Often they were also provided with free food, fuel, clothes, etc.; special medical care was probably not given. In the 16th and particularly the 17th century in a great many cities in the Netherlands—such as Amsterdam, Haarlem, Leiden, Delft, The Hague, Groningen—quite a number of 'hofjes' were built many of which still exist and are still inhabited by old people after having been renovated and modernised extensively. These 'hofjes' were mostly centrally located and by just passing a gate, the old person could enter into 'full life' again. Thus they were not shut off from the community in which they had been living before. By being grouped together in a 'hofje' some surveillance of their physical and mental health could be maintained.

Other charities were also beginning at the end of the Middle Ages for the poor, destitute and aged, who had no money for food and nowhere to live. These were mostly under the auspices of the church (first the Roman Catholic church and later the Protestant church.) Special buildings were equipped or built to take care of the sick, the poor, the aged and the vagabonds. These houses were called 'gasthuizen' (guesthouses). From this gasthuis—often also called hospitias— gradually developed the modern hospital. Some of the houses, e.g. the so-called 'Dyakony-

Huys' (Protestant poor relief board home) were specifically meant for the poor and the aged. Both the Catholic 'Heilige Geest' (Holy Ghost) organisation and (partly) its successor, the 'diakonie' (reformed poor relief board) worked as semigovernmental institutions and therefore had to take care of public relief of the poor. In the poor-houses (later also called workhouses, as the inmates had to work) the majority of the inmates was old. Often they were also ill and/or disabled, but generally not much medical care was offered (van der Leeden, 1956). The diseased and disabled formed a serious problem, mainly because there was insufficient accommodation for bedfast inmates. For example, there was generally no separation possible from those who had contagious disease. Gradually, from the 18th century the poor relief boards ordered the doctors in their charge to visit the home once or twice a week.

Some doctors had an interest in old age and the disease of old age. The famous Boerhaave (1668-1738) for example, advised an old ailing burgomaster to regain his vitality by just lying in bed between two young maidens. In the Dutch and Flemish arts of design we find only very few pictures of old sick people. Although several famous Dutch painters painted aging and old people (Rembrandt painted a series of self-portraits in the course of his own aging process; Franz Hals lived himself in an almshouse at Haarlem), the weakness, the dependency and the infirmity of both the very young and the old were seldom pictured. Quite well-known is a painting of an obese old man by Jacob Jordaens (1593-1678).

From two surgeons of the poor relief board home at Rotterdam in 1803 came the request to be permitted to do an autopsy on some old inmates who had died, 'to find out the disease and to be useful for the society'.

In the description of the Rotterdam home of the aged we learn that gradually in the 19th century some wards were assigned to ill (old) people and that at the end of that century an internal chief nurse and a few nurses were appointed. Thus in the same home, healthy and ill old people were still cared for together.

This combination continued in many homes built for the aged in the first half of the 20th century. The more seriously ill or handicapped old people were treated and nursed in the general (or mental) hospitals, the others in the old people's homes.

Before World War II several municipalities and private organisations built such mixed homes for healthy, ambulant, frail but not too ill or invalid old people in the Netherlands. Sometimes they were situated in central parts of towns and villages, but often they were in the suburbs or even isolated in parks, woods or fields (assuming that old people needed tranquillity and would enjoy the view of nature). Medical care was given by the person's own general practitioner or sometimes by a family doctor who was responsible for the health of all old people in the home.

The prevailing thought was that old people, if they should fall ill, should not be removed to other institutions (e.g. hospitals) if at all possible. Yet we see in the twenties and thirties the first nursing-homes come into existence. Often run by one or two (registered) nurses they offered nursing care in mostly small converted buildings (villas, etc.) Only very few especially designed nursing-homes were then built. The larger old people's homes had sections or departments, to which the real patients and invalids were moved once they could no longer care sufficiently for themselves.

After the war, specifically in the sixties, a new development in the institutional care system for certain types of ill old people occurred. While the general and mental hospitals continued to admit and treat mostly acutely ill old people these institutions showed much less interest in those with long-term disease or disability, often with multiple pathology. The hospitals became more and more specialised. This development made the hospitals ever more expensive. Since general practitioners are not permitted to work in general hospitals in the Netherlands, the specialists became more and more remote from the possibilities and difficulties of the aged in the community. Since these patients could not always be looked after by their relations and others in their own house and since old people's homes became more reluctant to admit them, the institute of the 'nursing home' began to develop. Churches and other charitable organisations and municipalities began to provide nursing-homes, run on a non-profit basis. Sometimes the sick funds would cover the costs, but more often this was not the case.

The financial basis of such institutions (often partly consisting of funds through the General Assistance Act) remained weak, until in 1968 the so-called General Special Sickness Expenses Insurance Act came into force. This Act, under which gradually more health provisions were offered, is of particular importance for the aged long-term sick. It provides exclusively (to all age-groups) for special costly or very prolonged treatment and/or nursing (for the physically and/or mentally handicapped, chronically ill, or mentally disturbed.) This Act does not take into account organisation, planning and coordination. It provides treatment in a 'recognised' nursing-home from the very first day if this is thought necessary. Later in this chapter more attention will be given to the nursing home.

Hospitals are mostly run on a non-profit basis, by private secular or religious organisations. There are also several hospitals run by the municipalities. The hospitals are independent, but they have in general to adhere to the prices approved by the central government. The same applies to nursing-homes (q.v.).

Although in general hospitals a high percentage (25% or more) of the patients is over 65 years of age, there has so far—with two exceptions—been no development of geriatric departments. To be clear, in the opinion of most 'geriatricians' in the Netherlands, the great majority of aged patients are not geriatric cases. Such a case exists particularly when invalidity, disability, helplessness and dependence on others threaten to occur after a disease or accident.

The absence of geriatric departments hampers the development of a medical specialty of geriatrics on its own. In the meantime, a sort of specialisation in geriatrics and medical care of the chronic sick has come into existence. In conclusion it may be said that in the last ten years or so, despite the absence of an official recognition of geriatrics, medical care for physically ill old people has developed to a high standard.

The development of medical care for mentally infirm old people has been the same in many respects as that of the physically infirm. A great deal of the accommodation in mental hospitals (up to one-third of the beds) was used for the elderly. They were cared for, but very little active treatment was given. In the fifties, however, a few medical doctors—psychiatrists and others—began to try a more active approach towards these patients. In a number of mental hospitals special geriatric departments were created, in which through various measures—such as drug treatment, physical, occupational and recreational therapy and sometimes through group psychotherapy—much is done to get the elderly patients discharged either to their own home, to an old persons' home, or to a specific nursing-home for mentally confused old people. The last is another important development in the medical care for the aged in the Netherlands. These specially designed nursing-homes began to come into existence after 1955. They concentrate, as do nursing-homes for the physically disabled, on active treatment. In the beginning the concept was that the two types of nursing-home should be quite separate institutions. Gradually this idea has changed. Although in general it is considered that serious physically and mentally ill old people should not be accommodated in the same rooms or wards—some experiments in mixing less seriously ill patients of both categories are proceeding. Some of these experiments are successful and the prevailing idea is now that a combined nursing-home may offer the best solution, provided that the units for the two types of patients are separated from one another.

THE PRESENT SITUATION

Primary health care

This type of care is also called 'first-echelon care' or 'first-line care' in the Netherlands.

(*a*) *At home:* In principle the following three persons are considered the main providers of primary care at home: the general practitioner, the district nurse (Dutch: wijkverpleegster) and the social worker. Of great importance also in the first-line are: the district nursing-aide, the home care provider (Dutch: gezinsverzorgster = caretaker of the family) and the home-help (Dutch: gezinshelpster = help of the family). In several cases, particularly for long-term patients the following people are also important: the pastor, the physiotherapist, the occupational therapist, the chiropodist, the friendly visitor (a Dutch term for this person doesn't exist, although sometimes the words 'vriendschappelijk huisbezoek' (friendly visiting) or 'vriendschappelijk bezoeker' (friendly visitor) may be used) and last but not least members of the family or other relatives of the sick or incapacitated (old) person, and—perhaps more in rural areas—the neighbours.

In Figure 3.1 an attempt is made to illustrate the relative importance of all these 'helpers'.

It is a good thing that in principle all these care providers do not help only and exclusively aged patients, but all long-term sick and disabled people who are at home. Only one kind of helper gives care more or less exclusively to the aged, that is the so-called 'bejaardenhelpster' (help of the aged). She (very rarely he) is a home-help, who has or may have had some additional information and instruction on how to deal with old people. Home-helps and helps for the aged, who are often key people in enabling old people to live independently in their own homes, are often women who work part-time, e.g. housewives in their 40s or 50s, who have no longer to run a large household themselves. Helps for the aged are allowed to assist old people as long as necessary, sometimes throughout several years. Home-help for younger people is mostly restricted to six weeks.

(*b*) *In clinics:* Primary care may also be given in so-called 'dienstencentra' (service centres), bureaux (clinics) for specialised services (for guidance on problems of life, of marriage, etc.), special clinics (mostly for tuberculosis, sometimes for venereal diseases, and, as an experiment, for cardiovascular diseases, but only very occasionally as a clinic for old people) and polyclinics.

These institutions generally act as secondary care providers, because people are referred to them after having been seen by their general

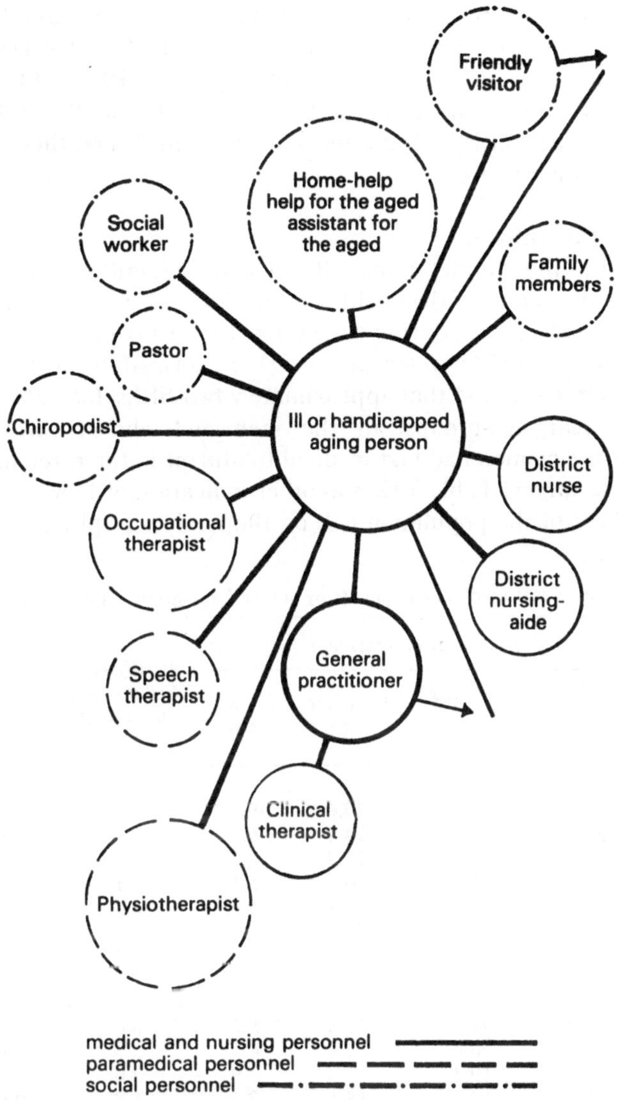

Figure 3.1 Members of the home-team responsible for health care of aging and old people.

practitioner, district nurse, or a social worker, i.e. by all or part of the 'home team'.

In particular polyclinics, which in the Netherlands are almost always attached only to a general hospital (sometimes to special hospitals such as for psychiatry, epilepsy, rehabilitation; and rarely to a nursing-home), are used by patients through reference by their GP. Occasionally polyclinics are used as primary care providers (e.g. for victims of (serious) accidents, for people with sight or hearing problems). So, although polyclinics may be considered as a form of extramural care, they are not identical to primary care.

The general practitioner

Together with the district nurse, the general practitioner is in the Netherlands the centre of the health care of the aged in the community.

In a nation-wide survey during the period 1955-1957 on the health of 3149 aged people (of 65 years and over), performed by 374 general practitioners it was found that approximately two-fifths, (35-45% in the various five-year age-groups) of the men and almost three-fifths (49-64%) of the women had had medical treatment in the three months preceding the survey. Table 3.12 is another indication of how much the older members of the population call on the services of physicians.

Table 3.12 Time of last medical treatment; by sex and age-groups; percentages

Age	*Last medical treatment*				*Hardly ever had medical treatment*	*Total*	
	3 months ago	*3 months-1 year ago*	*1-5 years ago*	*5 years ago*		*%*	*Abs*
Men							
65-69	39.4	18.5	23.6	9.7	8.8	100	351
70-74	35.7	22.2	24.1	9.4	8.6	100	406
75-79	45.1	19.8	21.2	7.3	6.6	100	410
80-84	43.2	25.5	20.1	5.1	6.1	100	294
85+	43.5	23.9	21.7	5.8	5.1	100	138
Total	41.0	21.5	22.3	7.8	7.4	100	1599
Women							
65-69	49.2	21.8	17.5	5.5	6.0	100	348
70-74	57.0	20.6	14.8	4.3	3.3	100	393
75-79	61.8	19.4	12.3	3.9	2.6	100	382
80-84	64.3	15.5	15.1	3.3	1.8	100	271
85+	59.8	19.1	12.5	5.3	3.3	100	152
Total	58.0	19.5	14.6	4.4	3.5	100	1546

The youngest group did so relatively least. This was especially the case for the women, for whom the percentage is nevertheless still 49 (for the men 39%). The distinct difference between the sexes on this point agrees approximately with the difference in their judgement of their own health It can also be seen that 15% (11-19%) of the men and 8% (5-12%) of the women had not asked for medical help during the preceding two years or more. About one-third of the men and one-fifth of the women had not consulted a doctor in the last year. It may thus be assumed that at least this fraction of the subjects had no chronic disease (or no severe form of such a disease) (van Zonneveld, 1961 b). Another figure supporting these data (Table 3.6) is that in the various five-year age groups 32-42% of the old men and 49-59% of the old women had regularly consulted a doctor.

In the mid-sixties it was already estimated that general practitioners spent 40% of their time on the 10-15% of their 'population' who were older than 64 years. Fuldauer (1966), a general practitioner, who examined all old people on his panel with the same questionnaire as used in the nation-wide survey, found that almost one-third of the men and two-thirds of the women in this practice were more or less regularly under his treatment. It appeared, that in the year before and in the year following his survey, some 60% of the men and 80% of the women had been seen by him. Since the population of the Netherlands will continue to age for the next twenty years or so (i.e. the percentage will increase), one must expect that the work of the general practitioner will become heavier.

According to the Dutch health insurance system people over 65 years of age can be members of a sick-fund, if they earn less than D.fl. 16 353 (April 1975) per year. They are then entitled amongst other things to free medical care by their general practitioners. There are about 4600 GPs in the Netherlands who are in charge of approx. 135000 old people living in their own house or in a residential home. In the residential homes, medical care is provided mostly by the old people's own GP, but in some homes one GP is in charge of all the residents.

Several family doctors make a habit of seeing the aged on their panel regularly, say each month, even if they have no complaints at all. This visit is sometimes used to check on certain points, e.g. blood pressure, depression and to give advice on diet, physical activity and social problems.

There is also a small number of GPs who run health clinics for the aged. General practitioners who run such health clinics get no extra pay for this work. They screen the old people who come at a special time, but have in general no complaints. Fuldauer (1966) advocated such a short mixed screening examination, which would take about seven minutes extra per day if all the old people in the practice were examined regularly at two-yearly intervals. Occasionally such a health clinic is not held in the general practitioner's home (the majority of Dutch general practitioners have consultation and/or treatment rooms in their own house), but in a health centre of the Cross societies for home care, or in a health centre run by GPs.

Besides their day-to-day care of the elderly and sometimes health screening, many GPs are also involved in medical examinations of old people, because most of the residential homes require such an examination before admission, in order to prevent too ill, too disabled old people entering.

A great number of general practitioners, whether or not they have special clinics for the elderly, give some time to health education of their old patients, e.g. with regard to diet, physical exercise (e.g. advice on participation in gymnastic clubs for old people), accident prevention, etc.

The district nurse

In the Netherlands by the end of the 19th century local societies had been founded by citizens (including general practitioners) to provide home care in case of illness and disability. These societies had a cross as an emblem. Later they were organised both on a national and a provincial level. The local societies have among their main tasks: home nursing, health education and the provision on loan of utensils for home-nursing. Almost all the communities in the Netherlands have at least one district nurse. It is estimated, on the basis of operational research, that up to 50% or 60% of her time is devoted to old people.

During the last few years in a number of areas nursing-aides have been appointed to assist the district nurse. The work of the former is to provide personal (nursing) care, such as: bathing and dressing the patient, bed-making, providing some movement 'therapy', etc.

POSTGRADUATE EDUCATION

Since GPs are so involved in medical care of the aged, there is a need for further education in this field. The Netherlands Institute for General Practitioners together with Professor Schreuder (Cahn *et al.*, 1973)), the pioneer of geriatrics in Holland, organised short courses for GPs. These were very well-attended, and are now offered at several places as postgraduate courses.

In the beginning mostly English books were used, sometimes translated into Dutch. Since 1960 and in particular in the last five years, several original Dutch books have been published, primarily for use by GPs, but also intended for medical students, nurses, physiotherapists and partly also for medical specialists. The first handbook in Dutch on old age, consisting mainly of chapters on medical problems appeared, however, in two parts, in 1948 and 1949. It was one of the first geriatric handbooks in Europe (Sleeswijk *et al.*, 1948, 1949).

In 1961 the present author edited a small volume on geriatrics (van Zonneveld *et al.*), which was followed by a much more comprehensive book *Medical Gerontology* in 1970 (van Zonneveld *et al.*). Several more books, e.g. on the gastrointestinal tract in old age (van Proosdij, 1966), on rehabilitation (Braadbaart *et al.*, 1971), on internal medicine (van Proosdij, 1972), a small *Vademecum on Geriatric Therapy* (Schouten and Rengelink, 1971) appeared. Schreuder, who was nominated as a special professor in gerontology at the University of Utrecht on behalf of the Netherlands Society for Gerontology, was honoured for his work in promoting geriatrics by a collection of his papers (Cahn *et al.*, 1973).

GENERAL PRACTITIONER RESEARCH

Research on geriatric problems has also been carried out by some general practitioners (usually those associated with nursing-homes). The following is a brief review.

Oostvogel (1968) studied 1678 persons who had entered their names on the waiting list for admission to a residential home in The Hague.

> 'Some 25% of prospects required no help; some 50% required help in self-care or domestic activities, while 4.5% required and received help in both self-care and domestic activities. Help was required but absent or insufficient for 18.6% of prospects.
>
> Help in self-care was most frequently provided by the marital partner, and next frequently by a visiting nurse. In prospects aged 85 and over requirements for help in self-care were five times as high as in those under 65. For domestic activities, requirements in the highest age-group were half again as high as in the youngest prospects'. . . .
> 'About 25% of prospects were suffering from conditions directly affecting stamina; nearly 25% had affections of the locomotor apparatus, nearly 20% were free from any affections. Male prospects showed a considerably lower incidence of affections of the locomotor apparatus than did female prospects. More than 50% of prospects in good mental condition were not or only slightly care-dependent; some 40% were care-dependent or seriously care-dependent; 4.5% were very seriously care-dependent. Corresponding percentages in prospects in unfavourable mental condition were 29.8, 59.6 and 10.6, respectively. In those with a less favourable mental condition, therefore, care dependence was considerably higher'. . . .

'Both in male and female prospects in favourable mental condition, there was a highly significant difference in care dependence between those living alone and those living in marriage; the married prospects were less care-dependent. No such difference was found in prospects who were in unfavourable mental condition'.

The social workers judged that admission could be postponed at least for some time for nearly 60% of prospects.

Welten (1968) carried out a two year longitudinal study on the 430 old people admitted into the general hospitals of the province of Zeeland on 31st January 1965. Some of his conclusions are:

1. One out of four old people, admitted or re-admitted to hospital, died in hospital within the year following the starting date. The flow through the general hospital, as far as aged patients are concerned, is therefore characterised by one death for every four patients.
2. At least one out of every four of the old people concerned in the investigation has to be considered chronically ill or infirm.
3. Those chronically ill old people, especially, slow down the flow through the hospital because their dismissal causes difficulties.
4. The lack of admission facilities in institutions outside the hospital is the main reason why dismissal is hampered. It was calculated that in fact one of every three old people would have to enter an institution after leaving hospital.
5. The 'silting up' of the general hospitals not only endangers the specific task of the general hospital as it exists at present, but also prejudices the recovery of the old people themselves.
6. The course of fitness, as well as the lack of room in institutions, certainly hampers a number of old people in their attempts to find a suitable environment after leaving hospital.
7. There are no indications that the results of the investigation can be considered characteristic for aged hospital patients exclusively. Only differences in degree seem to exist between aged hospital patients and all hospital patients taken together, and these can be attributed to the fact that with increasing age, a person's health gradually deteriorates.'

Welten concludes his summary as follows:

'Only often repeated assessments of the possibilities of assistance being given to old people in their localities and of the institutional facilities for old people, a strengthening of the contacts between the general hospital and the old people's welfare establishments, together with the creation of sufficient provisions, only these will make it possible for the hospital to discharge all patients quickly once they have recovered. If no suitable measures are taken, the sluice-gate function of the hospital will be adversely affected. The hospital would then have to start adapting itself to an increasing number of chronically ill and mentally disturbed old people.'

Leering (1968) studied the functional capacities of patients in 120 nursing-homes in the Netherlands.

'The following results were obtained from mentally normal patients:

1. A systematic arrangement of the activities of daily living recorded was discernible. Five ADL-levels can be distinguished, each of them containing one or more of the following ADL-functions: incontinence, eating, toilet function, dressing, bathing. There is a residual group of patients which could not be classified.
2. Incontinence occurs as an additional phenomenon at four levels, but is mostly encountered at the lowest two ADL-levels.
3. No correlation between sex and ADL-functions was encountered in this investigation.
4. A significant correlation was observed between ADL-levels and walking possibilities.
5. ADL-disorders show a significant correlation with the functional condition of the locomotor apparatus. The largest number of ADL-disorders per patient are seen in the group of paralyses and pareses. The group of contractures and/or restrictions of movement is characterised by a lower frequency of ADL-disorders per patient than the preceding group. Patients in the amputation group show the lowest incidence of ADL-disorders.

   As regards functional disorders of the sense organs the sensory disorders showed no clear-cut correlation with any ADL-level. Disorders of speech, on the other hand, were relatively more frequent at the lowest ADL-level and in the residual group.
6. There is a correlation between the category of affectations and the ADL-level. Patients with affectations of the CNS and patients in catabolic states have a significantly lower ADL-level than others. Internal affectations, with the exception of affectations of the cardio-vascular system and the lungs, show no correlation with ADL-level.
7. Only indirect correlations were found between number of ADL-disorders and age-group.
8. Pronounced correlations were found to exist between functional

disorders, affectations, age and evaluation of the possibility of reactivation. In the oldest age-group (85+), disorders of speech and paralyses/pareses show a significantly lower prevalence. This lower prevalence runs parallel with the relative decrease in the number of patients suffering from affectations of the CNS. There is a relative increase in the number of patients in the basic category 'internal affectations exclusively'.

9. The physician's assessment about the possibility of reactivation did not show any relationship with chronological age.

In the patients with mental disorders the following correlations could be observed:

1. The same systematic arrangement of ADL could be shown as was found in mentally normal subjects.
2. Incontinence occurs as an additional phenomenon at five levels and at each of these levels relatively more than in the mentally normal patients.
3. Every additional functional disorder of the locomotor or sensory apparatus causes the prevalence of a lower ADL-level than in the mentally normal group.
4. A pronounced correlation could be found between walking and the ADL. Patients with mental disturbances walk less frequently with walking aids than do mentally normal patients.
5. Every group of affectations gives rise to more ADL-disorders than in the mentally normal category.
6. Affectations of the CNS and particularly, affectations of the locomotor apparatus, occur significantly less often than in the mentally normal group.
7. The mentally disturbed patient is particularly vulnerable where his ADL are concerned and his chances of reactivation are small. The mentally disturbed patients in this investigation all suffer from an inexorable, progressive deterioration of their structuring capacities. Any aid ministered to these patients should be considered in this light.

The correlation between age, category of affectation and functional disorder can be regarded as the infrastructure of the ADL-function'.

Tonino (1969), a social geriatrician associated with a municipal health department, interviewed and thoroughly examined, with the help of others, a random sample of 400 old people. From the summary of his study the following is quoted:

'Of the 398 persons (two unknown)
—43 appeared to have no complaints;

—239 had minor complaints in one or more fields;
—116 had serious complaints in one or more fields.

In respect of 55 medical and biochemical questions an investigation was made in how far there existed an abnormality.

Out of the 398 persons (two unknown)
—7 appeared to have no abnormality at all;
—252 had at least one minor abnormality;
—139 had at least one serious abnormality.

However, out of the aged persons, who had no complaints, a comparatively large percentage appeared to have minor or serious abnormalities'. . . .

'Impotence for one or more activities of daily living functions was stated in the case of 67 out of the 400 persons investigated (16.8%), of whom 36 were slightly invalid, 11 moderately and 20 seriously invalid. As regards doing their own housekeeping 18% of the 400 persons examined was lightly unable, 26% moderately and almost 32% seriously unable'. . . .

'After the investigation a total opinion of the health condition was given. According to this integral opinion of health condition the 400 aged persons can be classified as follows:

	%
healthy	21
moderately healthy with curable abnormalities	48
moderately healthy with chronic abnormalities	16
seriously unhealthy	13
unfavourable prognosis	2

As in the case of health condition a total opinion was also given in regard to validity independence. According to this integral opinion of validity the 400 aged persons can be classified as follows:

	%
valid	67
moderately invalid with possibility of revalidation	11
moderately invalid of a chronic nature	13
seriously invalid	9

There is a clear relation between integral health and integral validity. However this does not mean, that all seriously or moderately unhealthy aged persons are to be considered as invalid. Out of 60 aged persons who were seriously unhealthy 31% was completely valid and 8% moderately invalid, but with a possibility of revalidation'. . . .

'The aged females appeared to be more in need of help by their family doctor than the males. The aged males needed more help by specialists than the females'. . . .

'The investigation showed that in medical as well as in social matters there is a big discrepancy betwee the objective need for help of the aged persons and the help actually received'.

Fennis and van Zonneveld (1973) undertook a large survey on the health and chronic conditions of people over 40 years of age in a city (Leiden) and a province (Friesland). Only a few data can be cited:

'Among the very old, institutionalisation on the indication of mental disorder occurs three times as often among women as among men, both in Leiden and in Friesland; the indication for admission to a nursing-home occurs 1½ times as often among women as among men, in both surveys.

In Leiden, almost twice as many admissions to homes for the aged are necessary for women than for men; in Friesland the difference is 20%. This may be due to the fact that Friesland has relatively more very old men and more very old married persons than Leiden, while furthermore it has more homes and a shorter waiting list, as a result of which admission is possible with less delay and selection is less strict. Also in Friesland, most administrators of homes for the aged still adhere to the policy of only admitting healthy old people.

As stated, the age group between 75 and 80 is only slightly larger than the group aged 80 years and above in Leiden, in Friesland and in fact in the Netherlands as a whole. The two age groups are therefore suitable for comparison in regard to the need for care. The very old need relatively 2½ to 3 times as many admissions as the 75 to 79 group; very old men 3 to 4 times and very old women about twice as often as the 75-79 group. Accordingly there is a considerable increase in the need for care from the younger to the older of these two groups. It would appear that 80 years is the 'turning point' at which institutionalisation very often becomes necessary, a fact that should be taken into account in the shaping of future policy.

Logically, married persons should need relatively less intramural care than those who are no(t) (longer) married. The need of the latter category is relatively 3 to 5 times as high. For aged married men the need for institutionalisation amounts to 4-5%, and for those who are unmarried or no longer married to 13-20%. For aged married women, the need lies between 5 and 6%, and for single females, widows and divorcees between 17 and 25%.

Among the aged, whatever the marital status, women need more institutional care than men.'. . .

'The need for beds in nursing-homes for the aged can only be reduced when the progress of conditions causing invalidity can be arrested. Extension of extramural care facilities has little or no influence on the need for admission to a nursing-home. But when will they be extended? It is perhaps not impossible that in the not too distant future, euthanasia will be legalised. This may then influence the need for beds, particularly in nursing-homes for the aged mentally handicapped. The number of beds for aged mental patients will be increased (from the 1969 figure of almost 9000 beds) to 13 750 before 1980, enough for almost 0.9% of the aged population. Between 1960 and 1980, demographic alterations are expected to cause an increase in institutionalisation of 0.4%, which implies the institutionalisation of an additional 6000 aged persons above the 1960 requirements, or an additional 2000 above the 1970 requirements, estimated at approximately 30 000. By 1980, the need for beds for mentally handicapped aged persons will be 2 to 3 times higher than currently alleged.

Under the influence of demographic changes alone, the proportion of the aged needing admission to homes for the aged will increase from 6.4% in 1960 to 7.3% in 1980. The proportion of the aged living in homes for the aged has been 8% since 1968 and will be about 10% in 1975. Accordingly, a proportion of 10% would not appear to be too low, particularly when more special housing projects for the aged will have been realised.'

Finally, a study by the medical director of a nursing-home Merkus (1974) in 364 patients admitted in 1968-9 to a nursing-home may be mentioned.

'78.0% of the resident patients and 35.5% of the newly-admitted patients were diagnosed as long-term patients. Discharge was considered likely in respectively 12.5% and 42.3% and death occuring within six months, in respectively 9.4% and 24.2%.

69.8% of the resident patients and 26.9% of the newly-admitted patients were still cared for after six months. 9.0% and 34.3% respectively had been discharged and in 21.2% and 38.7% respectively death had occurred.'. . .

'In the group of newly-admitted patients to our nursing-home females are over-represented in comparison with the sex-ratio of the overall population. We have made it likely that the fact that females tend to be—more often than males—single, without children and living alone must be one of the reasons for their being over-represented. Another explanation can be found in the higher morbidity among female patients as compared with male patients. This difference especially manifests itself in locomotor and mental disorders, which are both more frequent among female patients than male. Because these affections often occur in the group of newly-admitted patients, it is likely that these differences in morbidity are among the causes of female over-representation.'. . .

'The situation after six months after admission is more favourable for female patients than male, independent of a number of other relevant factors.

There is no correlation between age-groups and the situation after six months in the various categories of dependency.

The patients who before their admission lived alone, show a more favourable pattern in the course of the illness than the other patients, independent of a number of other relevant factors.'

These few examples may demonstrate that particularly among GPs, or former GPs who have become medical directors of nursing-homes or social geriatricians, a good deal of gerontological research of a socio-medical nature has been carried out. Less has appeared on the clinical side.

HOSPITAL CARE

General hospitals

With a very few exceptions, general hospitals in the Netherlands have no separate geriatric departments. One of the exceptions, the geriatric department in the general hospital 'Zonnestraal' (a former sanatorium) at Hilversum was founded by Professor Schreuder. Special geriatric hospitals are not favoured at all although special geriatric nursing-homes are very common.

According to standard procedures, old people are admitted just as younger ones. However, aged patients with chronic disease or disability are often not accepted but referred to a nursing-home. In principle they are first seen at the polyclinics. The departments of internal medicine and surgery in particular deal with large numbers of the over 65s. They are examined and treated as other, younger, patients. Special emphasis is now given to maintaining mobility and to keeping the old person as briefly as possible in the hospital.

Some general hospitals, among them university hospitals, are now considering the creation of special geriatric departments, to concentrate more on the problems and potentials of aged patients, to educate and train doctors, nurses and paramedical personnel in dealing with the elderly and to offer better possibilities for clinical geriatric research. Geriatrics is not a recognised medical speciality in the Netherlands at present—as has been stated before—but several doctors have specialised themselves, training partly in foreign geriatric units. Geriatricians, who are now working mostly as physicians in nursing-homes, besides needing experience in general medicine, psychiatry and neurology and rehabilitation medicine, require a great deal of social medicine.

The financing of hospital treatment of old people is regulated in the same way as for younger persons. More than 80% of all old people in the Netherlands are members of a sick-fund, mostly on a voluntary basis, although sometimes—if they are still working and have an income under a certain level—compulsory. To be a voluntary sick-fund member a person of 65 or older must also be under a certain income level (as from April 1975 under D.fl. 16 353 a year). According to the income level he pays a certain monthly premium; under certain conditions their family-members are also fully insured. Premiums in D.fl. are as follows:

Married persons		*Unmarried persons*	
Income (annual)	*Premium (monthly)*	*Income (annual)*	*Premium (monthly)*
0-11 628	18.20	0-8311	18.20
11 628-11 966	54.40	8311-11 628	36.20
11 966-12 638	72.40	11 628-12 638	72.40
12 638-14 496	90.50	12 638-16 353	90.50
14 496-16 353	126.75		

To compare these figures: the monthly state old-age pension is for a single person: D.fl. 665.50 for a married couple: D.fl. 943.00 (as from 1st April 1975).

The provisions for the voluntary insured (which includes most of the aged) are the same as for the compulsory insured. They consist, amongst other things, of full medical treatment by their own general practitioner; by a specialist (including polyclinics at general hospitals) or treatment in the polyclinics of a university hospital; dental care (under certain conditions), medicaments (with certain exceptions), physical therapy (within certain limits), orthopaedic shoes, protheses, hearing-aids, glasses, etc. transportation, other provisions and examinations, treatment and nursing care in the cheapest (common) class of a hospital (including mental hospitals and sanatoria), but only for one year per admission (treatment includes physiotherapy, occupational therapy, etc., in other words all the provisions a modern hospital should give). If the patient has to stay in hospital longer than a year, this will be paid for according to the General Exceptional Medical Expenses (Compensations) Act.

Most of those old people who are not in a sick-fund, have a private sickness insurance which provides them with free or almost free hospital care.

In general, hospital admission is not a financial catastrophe, neither for the old person himself nor for his relatives.

The general practitioner receives a *per capita* fee for those who are in the sick-fund system (somewhat less than 70% of the total population). Those who are in a private insurance system, or who are not insured at all, pay separately for each item of service. The *per capita* fee of the sick-fund system is (1973) (up to 1800 patients on the list): D.fl. 29.76 plus 17.05 for costs, i.e. 46.81 per patient per year. For all patients beyond 1800 the figures are: D.fl. 29.76 + 1.64 for costs = 31.40 per patient per year (£1 is approx. D.fl. 5.75).

Mental hospitals

Although many beds in mental hospitals are occupied by old people, with newer methods of treatment their number is slowly diminishing. The conditions under which they are admitted have already been mentioned under the section 'General Hospitals.'

Several mental hospitals have now geriatric departments, where psychiatrists trained in psycho-geriatrics, actively treat mentally unfit old people. Several of these hospitals also have an observation department, mostly in connection with a municipal health service. Here acutely confused old people are first examined, internally, neurologically and psychologically—and treated, before further steps are taken (such as admission to a mental hospital, a general hospital, a nursing-home, etc.)

Some mental hospitals also have day-hospital accommodation.

Day hospitals

General hospitals in Holland do not have a day hospital; some mental hospitals and nursing-homes, however, do (called then: day-nursing). They pay roughly the same role as day hospitals in Great Britain: prevention of admission to a hospital or nursing-home, after-care for those discharged patients, who are still incapable of living independently in their own surroundings or in old people's homes and sometimes as an institution providing temporary relief for the family, or for intensive treatment and rehabilitation.

Experiments with night hospitals for the elderly, where an old person (e.g. mentally confused) is accepted only for the night have not been tried as yet.

Nursing-homes

Although this institution has already been mentioned several times in this chapter, some more attention may be given to it, since nursing-homes provide the most specific intramural care for the aged sick in Holland. There now exists (1974) roughly 33 000 beds in these institutions, of which more than 9000 are for mentally impaired old people.

A nursing-home for physically ill old people is an institution for patients who do not need continuous specialist (medical) care but who do need expert medical treatment, continuous nursing and general care, usually following examination and treatment in a general hospital.

Whatever name this sort of institution has in other countries there clearly exists in Holland the need for an institution coming between hospital and residential or old folk's home. According to extensive surveys undertaken by the author and in collaboration with others in the Netherlands there exists a need for nursing-homes for the physically ill for at least 2% of the aged and for about 1.5% of moderately mentally confused old people. Perhaps these percentages are on the high side but it is clear that a good system of nursing-homes of both types will relieve general and mental hospitals of an important part of the burden of long-term care of chronic sick and disabled old people.

Nursing-homes also serve as final stations for those who remain chronically ill and disabled, cannot be cared for elsewhere and therefore stay until their death in that sort of institution; long-stay wings therefore form part of the nursing-home.

Another absolute necessity is that nursing-homes have strong formal functional relations with general and/or mental hospitals and also with a number of old people's homes.

Unfortunately only in a minority of cases are these bonds already ensured. There is, however, a growing tendency in several cities to have or to create central referral systems, so that the patient comes into the right bed.

From an organisational point of view hospitals, nursing-homes, day hospitals, out-patients clinics, health and welfare clinics or service centres (see below) and possibly residential homes and the whole array of extramural services should indeed form one system of care. In Holland the term 'closed circuit' is then used.

Such a system can very well also serve other age-groups, particularly the chronic sick and disabled among them.

From the above it may be clear that the term 'nursing-home' is not very appropriate. It may be repeated that a major function of this institution is to bring sick and disabled old people back to normal, community life. Several nursing-homes in Holland are therefore also called 'geriatric clinic' or 'reactivation centre'.

The size of these institutions is on an average of 150-175 beds for the physically impaired and 60-70 for the mentally impaired (in which case they are combined homes). One other point should also be made clear; the nursing-home is not exclusively for the aged, although in the homes for the physically sick and disabled more than 80%, even 90%, are over the age of 65.

In the beginning the tendency was to build separate nursing-homes for the physically ill and for the mentally disabled old people. During the last few years however, a combined building is preferred, although the two departments remain generally well separated.

COMMUNITY CARE

In Holland as in other countries, the fact is often overlooked that care of the aged, including social care, brings involvement with physical and/or mental disease and disability. Sometimes in the network of community care too little attention is paid to this important aspect. Although many social services are provided, the causal health factor is not considered sufficiently. On the other hand it must be stated that sometimes the medical model gets too much emphasis.

In the preceding paragraphs, dealing with primary care, something has already been said about community care. Therefore, only a brief review will be given here.

Health care is provided in the first place by the GP and the district nurse and in later stages if necessary by specialists, general and mental hospitals, nursing-homes for physically ill long-term patients and nursing-homes for mentally infirm old people. Some of these institutions have day-treatment and nursing centres. In some of the bigger cities the municipal health services have departments for social geriatrics, which for instance control or mediate in the admission of old people to certain intra- and extramural facilities and services. Mention has also been made of the clinics which a small number of GPs hold to provide preventive services, e.g. a short examination and screening of healthy old people on their panel.

Housing. For those who are no longer able to do their housekeeping (mostly because of impaired health or of general weakness and frailty) there is the possibility of being admitted into an old people's home. Together these provide (1974) more than 130 000 beds. Also special small dwellings are built for the aged (and for younger handicapped persons), which are easier to use, clean, etc. (These small houses generally are connected by telephone or alarm-bell system to a central post). In the 1970s about 13 000 of such units are being built each year; there are now about 80 000 of them.

Local services. Various services are given to old people who because of poor health or frailty cannot undertake certain tasks, such as cooking, shopping, cleaning. These include meals-on-wheels, home-helps or special assistants of the aged, etc. A certain centralisation of the various services and provisions is now under way in the so-called service centres. Provision of these centres is stimulated, amongst other things by subsidies from the central and local authorities.

It should be said that there is still in many instances a lack of coordination and cooperation. This is partly caused by a shortage of manpower in certain services and/or regions. To help in meeting this problem home-helps have been permitted for several years past to work as part-timers and for an indefinite time, for old people. Another solution may be to bring in many more volunteers; among them the healthy aged themselves.

EDUCATION

Medical practitioners

1. In the medical curriculum of some (but not yet all) medical faculties special lectures or courses are given to medical students. At Leiden University for instance, second-year students attend a four-day course on (medical) gerontology and third and fourth-year students attend a three-day course in geriatrics. The courses are not compulsory; in the examinations of other disciplines, however, a few questions are included on gerontology and geriatrics. Moreover, visits to nursing-homes and old people's homes are included in the practical part of social medicine. The Institute of Social Medicine at Leiden University, provides also for lectures on social gerontology and workshops on the health care of the aged.

The Medical faculty at Utrecht offers a number of afternoon bedside teaching lectures at the geriatric department of a hospital.

The Institute for Social Medicine at Nijmegen offers to many students an internship of two to four weeks in a nursing-home.

These are a few examples of how medical faculties are gradually starting to interest their students in gerontology and geriatrics.

2. Postgraduate courses in gerontology and geriatrics as such do not yet exist in the Netherlands, but recently two courses started for physicians working in nursing-homes. Such courses are not full-time, but present a series of lectures and demonstrations in the course of a year. Some geriatric departments and nursing-homes also offer an internship in geriatrics.

It should be added that short courses for general practitioners and specialists are also provided at two university cities. These are particularly popular with general practitioners who spend a great deal of their daily work in providing care for the elderly.

Nurses

In the renewed education and training of registered nurses much attention is now paid to the care of the chronic sick and the aged. In the additional training for district nurses particular emphasis is laid on various aspects of health care of the aging and the aged.

There are some special courses for registered hospital, nursing-home and district nurses, in gerontology and geriatrics.

Nursing-aides

Until about ten years ago no specific education and recognition existed for these health workers. Since then the official profession of 'ziekenverzorgster' (caretaker of the patient) has been established. These nursing-aïdes get an officially recognised two year theoretical and practical full-time education and training to assist registered nurses. But the work of nursing-aides is mainly focused at nursing care of the long-term and aged sick. So in all nursing-homes and in many old people's homes one can find these women working for the benefit of ill and disabled old people.

Special manuals are written for the training of nursing-aides in geriatrics (e.g. Akkerman, 1973).

Other professions

The most important is the 'bejaardenhelpster' (help for the aged), who works mostly in old people's homes but also in the community. They can offer simple nursing-care, but are mainly involved in general (household) care. These helps for the aged have also an officially recognised two-year theoretical and practical education and training and have—like the nursing-aides—special badges and certificates.

The 'gezinshelpsters' (helps of the family) also offer a great deal of domestic care to the aged.

Matrons of old people's homes can enrol in part-time courses and recently full-time courses have been introduced. In the training of physiotherapists, occupational therapists, social workers, etc., of course, some attention is given to the aspects of care for the elderly.

Liaison and coordination

Relations between the various care-giving organisations are not always optimal and indeed are quite insufficient. The need for combined action, however, is gradually becoming apparent. Various patterns are possible.

1. In the bigger cities the municipal health departments provide a certain coordination, particularly when municipal services (hospitals, nursing-homes, old people's homes, district nurses, social workers, transportation, etc.) are involved. Sometimes the municipal health department forms part of a so-called central point for reference and admission.

2. In other instances in certain towns or villages local councils or committees for the aged, which are trying to coordinate all the services an old person needs, see to it that the required services are indeed provided. Sometimes they may use scoring systems, but these can only work well when all intra- and if possible extramural services cooperate. This means that local (or sometimes regional) public authority and private institutions and other services are brought together and voluntarily decide to cooperate fully. One of the major results of such a cooperation is the realisation of a central point (committee or office) where with the help of the scoring-system each person in need of some kind of care is actually provided with that care, particularly institutional care.

In various places scoring-systems have been partly tried out for several years, which give points (scores) for various factors, as age, isolation, grade of disability, nearness of family members, etc. According to the number of points allocation is made to the type of care needed.

3. More and more centres for provision of various services ('diensten centra') already referred to, play the role of coordinating body. Although the government in 1970 published a memorandum on old people's care (which has since been revised) and paid much attention to

coordination and liaison of services, in still too many instances this most important aspect of (health) care of the aged is underdeveloped.

Mention may also be made of a type of community service, the *health assessment* of the aged, in which full examination may be possible on an occasional basis. The big question is, of course, whether such periodic examinations are really necessary, since so many old people are already seeing their general practitioner regularly.

Another possibility is the multiphasic screening (e.g. on weight, height, blood pressure, blood haemoglobin, eye-ball pressure, urine (protein, sugar and sediment), eventually ECG, hearing and vision). In some instances GPs, mostly with the help of district nurses, do perform such screenings. Even health clinics for the elderly are proposed and exist in some places.

The same question remains, however, whether such screenings and such health clinics really add to the *full* well-being of the aged. In general it may be said that, in spite of various demands by the aged or others, there is much doubt as to the real value of such provisions. Fuldauer (cited above) therefore advocates that each GP should an old person so request, follow the examination for the presenting complaint, with some quick questions and investigations which on the average should prolong the consultation no more than ten minutes. In fact, several GPs and also some specialists try to get a deeper insight into the health situation of their patient. But this is as yet not a well-established procedure. Much more experimentation is still needed to decide this issue.

THE FUTURE

In looking at the present situation, opinions have been expressed as to how this situation should be improved for the benefit of the elderly. Therefore, it suffices to summarise a few points:

1. Among nursing-home doctors and some general practitioners as well as among a limited number of specialists there is a wish to make geriatrics a recognised medical speciality. It remains to be seen whether this development will indeed occur.

2. In the meantime several hundreds of doctors have made themselves specialists in the care of the aged and chronic sick.

3. In the medical curriculum as well as in the training and education of other workers in the health care of the aged, more and more

attention will be paid to gerontology and geriatrics. Also many more postgraduates courses will be offered.

4. It is uncertain whether many general hospitals will have geriatric departments in the future. But it is certain that more medical, nursing and social attention will be paid to elderly patients. Mental hospitals, which have in many cases already geriatric departments, will be more ready to continue creating such departments.

5. The nursing-home system, as existing in the Netherlands, will be further expanded, particularly for mentally impaired old people.

6. On the other hand, not so many homes for the aged will be built since the emphasis will be on keeping the aged, even in the case of illness and disability, in their own surroundings, preferably in their own house.

7. Therefore, community services for the aged will be greatly expanded. Unfortunately lack of manpower (and of money) will hamper this development.

8. A great role will be given to the service-centres in the provision of community services and in their coordination and liaison.

As a whole, it seems the future development of health care for the aged in the Netherlands will in most respects *not* differ much from the development in other Northern and Western European countries.

Final remark

The foregoing is not, of course, a complete picture of the situation and evolution of medical care for the elderly in the Netherlands. Many examples of already existing provisions and developments were not mentioned. It is always better to stay in a country for a certain time to become really knowledgeable about what is actually going on. It can be said, however, that although much is still lacking in the care for the aged in this country (and that refers particularly to the general attitude towards the oldest generation), a good deal is being done for their benefit.

It may be hoped that this evolution will go on, so that in the 21st century to be an older citizen in the Netherlands means no differentiation in any aspect of attention and care as compared with other age-groups.

References

Akkerman, H. P. (1973). *Geriatre (Geriatrics)* (Leiden: *Spruyt, van Mantgem and De Does*)

Braadbaart, S. *et al.* (1971). *Reactivering van Bejaarden. (Rehabilitation of the Aged*] (Leiden: Stafleu)

Cahn, L. A., Munnichs, J. M. A. and Schouten, J. (1973). *20 Jaar Geriatrie.* (*20 Years of Geriatrics; a Choice from the Publications by Prof. dr. J. Th. R. Schreuder*). (Deventer: van Loghum Slaterus)

Fennis, H. W. J. M. (1973). *Medische Demografie van Bejaarden; Bevolking, Sterfte, Ziekte en Invaliditeit (Medical Demography of the Aged; Population, Mortality, Morbidity and Invalidity).* (Thesis) (Leiden: Ned. Inst. Praev. Geneesk. TNO)

Fennis, H. W. J. M. and van Zonneveld, R.J. (1966-1970). *The Chronically Ill and Their Needs, 5 mimeographed reports.* (Leiden: Ned. Inst. Praev. Geneesk. TNO)

Fuldauer, A. E. (1966). *Bejaardenonderzoek in een Huisartspraktijk. (Health Examination of Old People in a General Practice).* (Thesis) (Hengelo: Insulinde)

Leeden, C. B. van der (1956). *De Ontwikkeling van Diakoniehuis tot Gemeentelijk Tehuis voor Ouden van Dagen te Rotterdam (The Development from Poor Relief Home into Municipal Home for the Aged at Rotterdam).* Rotterdam

Leering, C. (1968). *Gestoord Menselijk Functioneren. (Disorders of Human Functions)* (Thesis) (Nijmegen: Dekker en van de Vegt)

Mast, F. A. C. de, Remmerswaal, P. W. M. and Munnichs, J. M. A. (1972). *Atlas van de Ouder Wordende Nederlandse Bevolking. (Atlas of the Ageing Population of the Netherlands*) (Deventer: van Loghum Slaterus)

Merkus, J. W. F. M. (1974). *Verpleegtehuispatienten. (Patients in Nursing-homes)* (Thesis Nijmegen)

Oostvogel, F. J. G. (1968). *Verzorgingsbehoeften van Bejaarden. (Needs of the Aged for Care)* (Thesis) (Nijmegen: Dekker en van de Vegt)

Proosdij, C. van (1966). *Het Maag-darm Kanaal bij Bejaarden. (The Gastro-intestinal Tract in the Aged).* (Leiden: Stafleu)

Proosdij, C. van (1972). *Bejaarde Patienten. (Aged Patients)* (Leiden: Stafleu)

Schouten, J. and Rengelink H. (1971). *Vademecum Therapie Geriatrie. (Vademecum Therapy in Geriatrics)* (Amsterdam-Brussel: Agon Elsevier)

Sleeswijk, J. G. *et al.* (1948, 1949). *De Ouderdom van Geneeskundig Standpunt Beschouwd. (Old Age from the Medical Point of View)* Manual in 2 vol. (Amsterdam: Kosmos)

Tonino, F. J. M. (1969). *Bejaarden Thuis. (Old People at Home)* (Thesis Nijmegen)

Welten, J. B. V. (1968). *Bejaarden in Ziekenhuizen. (Old People in*

Hospitals) (Thesis) (Nijmegen: Dekker en van de Vegt)
Zonneveld, R J. van(1954). *Gezondheidsproblemen bij Bejaarden. (Health Problems in the Aged)* (Thesis) (Assen: Royal van Gorcum)
Zonneveld, R. J. van (ed.) (1961 a). *Geriatrie (Geriatrics).* (Assen: Royal van Gorcum)
Zonneveld, R. J. van (1961 b). *The health of the Aged.* (Assen: Royal van Gorcum)
Zonneveld, R. J. van (ed.) *et al.* (1970). *Medische Gerontologie. (Manual: Medical Gerontology*), (Assen: Royal van Gorcum)

CHAPTER FOUR

The United States of America

Isadore Rossman and
Irene Mortenson Burnside

HISTORY

The health care system in the USA is historically characterised by inequities which especially affected the poor and the elderly. To account for this prior to the landmark of Medicare legislation, one must point to the socio-economic origins and resultant cultural attitudes long dominant in the USA. In addition to the early 19th centure Jeffersonian philosophy that that government governed best which governed least, there were reinforcements from a exuberant *laissez faire* capitalism. This resulted in a philosophy whose basic tenet was that every man was on his own and that he who could not purchase desirable material goods or medical services had only himself to blame. This viewpoint was strengthened by the numerous examples of the acquisition of wealth afforded by a pioneering and vertically mobile society. In this land of opportunity the poor, both young and old, were regarded as self-generated failures in life's struggles. It is in this context that one must retrospectively judge the gross inadequacy of medical care and the almost uncountable episodes of man's inhumanity to man. An example of the latter were the notorious county poorhouses. These were domiciliary structures operated at the 'pinch-penny' level, designed for the care of the poor who were generally the disabled elderly. Inmates lived in large dormitories, subsisted on the cheapest food and received negligible medical care. Yet with all of their demeaning features, these were settings thought not unfit for the elderly poor.

Because of the well-known associations between aging, chronic illness and poverty the aged had always contributed a considerable percentage to the medically indigent population. As financial reserves ran out they fell into the charitable sector of hospital and medical care. The sick elderly thus supplied a hard core to the clinic and the in-hospital ward populations. The wards were traditionally dormitory-like facilities, not uncommonly with one to two dozen patients, if not more, in an open setting. Clinic and ward were in striking contrast to the private offices and private pavilions in which the well-to-do were treated. Essentially this produced a two-tier system of care which was quite characteristic of American medical practice throughout more than the first half of the 20th Century. The tiers were defined by economic considerations; the ability to pay the fee. Needless to say, the well-to-do elderly were able to enjoy private facilities including private psychiatric rather than state mental hospitals.

True, 'ward medicine' was not necessarily inferior to 'private medicine' at the better teaching hospitals, because ward patients might be seen by a team of physicians rather than a solo practitioner. Particularly during the years when the various subspecialties were emerging, such team medicine sometimes functioned at an inherently better diagnostic and therapeutic level. However, in a majority of hospitals, including the municipal hospitals built for the indigent, patients did in fact receive variable and often inadequate or hurried treatment. Another major defect was that the ward patient had no doctor of his own to whom he could turn for information, reassurance or continuity. The charity system of medicine, both in and out of hospital, was based on the concept of no fee or a sliding scale of fees. Though this could solve blatant emergencies requiring hospitalisation, ambulatory care suffered. Most private practitioners avoided this group of patients except in clinics, which were often discouragingly crowded. There is no doubt that this care structure cut down on many desirable or necessary opportunities for the patient to consult with a physician.

Even the middle class elderly had cause for apprehension. Compulsory retirement from industry often meant losing hospitalisation insurance supplied by employers. Because the elderly represented a high risk group, it was difficult, if not impossible, for many of them to purchase hospital insurance. Major medical or catastrophe insurance even with a large deductible, were virtually prohibitive in cost. The problems were compounded by the rising cost of medical care which, throughout the fifties and sixties, became the most runaway item in the cost of living index. As noted by Shanas in her 1962 survey, about half of older people said that they would be unable to meet substantial charges for medical care out of their own resources. She also noted that, 'The possibility of an extended illness is the greatest single threat to the peace of mind of the elderly'. Though a pension system, called Social Security, for elderly retirees had been set up in 1935, the amounts were essentially supplemental, continued to be eroded by inflation and contained no provisions for medical care payments.

Prior to the 1966 enactment of Medicare, there had been a number of proposals for solving the financial aspects of medical care. The Murray-Wagner-Dingell Bill (1948) was addressed to the needs of the entire population, not the 65 and over group alone. The bill proposed a national health insurance system to be financed by payroll taxes and administered by the Federal Government. It was backed by President Harry S. Truman, was lobbied against by the AMA (American Medical Association) and other interests and was narrowly defeated in the House of Representatives. Thus, almost two decades elapsed before insurance legislation was enacted. Passage of Medicare occurred in part because its benefits were limited to the elderly who were recognised as belonging to a particularly hard hit group.

Medicare

Basically Medicare legislation set up a form of 'major medical', hospital and medical insurance. The final bill contained many compromise features including one made necessary by the AMA's stand which provided for 'customary fees' to be paid to the physician. Also, to cut costs, some troublesome deductible features were introduced. The hospitalisation feature (Part A) is financed in large measure by a 1% tax on salaries, plus some contribution from general tax funds. Part B of the programme is financed through a voluntary monthly contribution by the insuree. This is the 'supplementary medical insurance', which pays for the doctor's bills, in or out of hospitals, plus a number of other expenses.

Monthly contributions have increased several times since 1966, because of rising costs. Also, the 'deductible' for hospitalisation, payable by the patient, has increased. As of the present writing, the major provisions of Medicare are the following:

1. Part A, the hospital insurance uses as a base, a 'benefit period', a period of time defined by a hospitalisation. The first benefit period consists of sixty consecutive days either in a hospital or in a hospital followed by a stay in a skilled nursing facility. The next benefit period begins when the patient has been out of a facility for sixty consecutive days. Under Part A, the patient is entitled to bed care in a hospital for upto ninety hospital days in each benefit period. The first $92 of hospital charges are payable by the patient. From the sixty-first and through the ninetieth day, the hospital insurance pays for all covered services except

for $23 a day. Also covered is care in a psychiatric facility, but with a life-time restriction of 190 days.

2. Part B, the supplementary medical insurance (SMI) is paid for at the rate of $6.70 per month, generally as a deduction from the individual's social security income. The following are covered: (1) doctor's services (2) out-patient hospital services (3) home-health services (4) medical services and supplies (5) physical therapy and (6) speech pathology services. There is a $60 deductible charge for these, payable by the patient. SMI pays 80% of the 'reasonable charges' for additional covered services after the first $60. There is a number of exclusions. For example, Part B does not pay for tests given as part of a routine check-up, or eye refractions for the purpose of fitting or changing eye-glasses, for immunisations, or hearing examinations for prescribing, fitting or changing hearing aids. Nor are important items such as prescription drugs, hearing aids, eye-glasses, false teeth or orthopaedic shoes covered. Another curious exclusion under Medicare is the first three pints of blood received in a benefit period, either in the hospital, or as an out-patient. The jumble of deductibles and exclusions was obviously intended to keep down the costs of the insurance programme. But as will be noted later, they have led to complicated book-keeping and to financial difficulties for some of the impoverished elderly.

Medicaid

In recognition of the financial problems faced by the medically or socially indigent of all ages, a Medicaid system was also set up. Medicaid is essentially a welfare rather than an insurance system and requires proof of need. The costs are paid for by state and local authorities in conjunction with grants from the Federal Government. Its chief application is in covering the various deductibles and especially for nursing-home care, the costs of which may be astronomical. Most, but not all, of the states have Medicaid legislation. The rules for qualification vary from state to state as do the amounts that Medicaid will pay for such items as a physician's service. Medicaid may thus be a paradoxical jumble of local reimbursement methods, illustrated by the fact that New York City will pay $6 for a physician's home visit and $20 for a nurse's home visit, the latter payable to the Visiting Nurse Service.

Unlike Medicare, therefore, Medicaid may pay distinctly less than prevailing fees, requires separate billing and is sometimes enmeshed in red tape. As a result, many physicians have decided not to accept Medicaid patients, including that small group over 65 who have not elected to purchase the SMI. In short, the two-tier system alluded to previously still remains, though fortunately the bulk of the elderly are now in the upper tier.

DIMENSIONS OF THE PROBLEM

A few highlights concerned with the aging population of the USA are the following figures which were extracted from a report of the Administration on Aging in February 1973: Every tenth American is over 65; almost 21 million. The figure will rise to 25 million by 1985. Every day approximately 4000 Americans become 65, 3000 aged 65+ die, with a net increase of approximately 1000 a day or over 350 000 a year. More than 1.5 million are 85 or over. The 1971 *per capita* health care cost for older Americans came to $861, almost three and a half times the amount spent for younger persons. Of this, $410 was for hospital care, $144 for physicians' services, $34 for other professional services, $87 for drugs, $151 for nursing-home care and $36 for miscellaneous items. 68% of the costs came from public programme resources. The ratio of women to men in the 65+ group is 139 to 100 with a total of roughly 12 million as compared to 8 million. Seven out of every ten older persons live in family settings; one-quarter live alone or with relatives; 4.3 million or 22% of the elderly were living in households with incomes below the official poverty level. Only one in twenty lives in an institution.

Medicare financial contributions to the medical structure are pointed up by the figures for 1972 from the Social Security Administration: There were 6.4 million hospitalisation claims for a total of 74 million days of care, approximately 11.7 days per claim. The total for hospitalisation amounted to over $7 billion with 76% reimbursed by Medicare. For the same period there were almost 52 million physicians' claims for a total of $3 billion, with 73% of this reimbursed.

MEDICAL PRACTICE CONSIDERATIONS

Though some obstacles and financial difficulties still remain, as will be discussed later, Medicare legislation has provided virtually unimpeded access to hospital and doctor for the bulk of the elderly population. For illustration, one might consider an elderly patient, who in a given year has need only for ambulatory services. He may consult an ophthalmologist for ocular problems, an internist for control of various medical disorders, perhaps a radiologist for X-rays and conceivably other specialists. If the doctors involved are willing to accept 'assignment' and the first $60 has been paid by the patient, then each doctor submits a bill on Medicare forms and is directly paid 80% of the allowable fee for his service. In some parts of the country where doctors have generally decided not to accept assignment, the patient may instead pay the fees charged to each doctor as he goes along. At various intervals, or even at the end of the year, the paid-for bills and covering Medicare forms are sent by the patient to the fiscal intermediary for Medicare. The allowable fees for the physician's services are totalled up, $60 is subtracted and the patient is reimbursed for 80% of the remainder. It is apparent that even with the supplementary medical insurance, the patient must needs pay $75.60 per year through his monthly premiums, plus a deductible of $60. But he may well be financially liable for the 20% of the allowable fee, or more, if the doctor's fee is higher than allowed. Similar considerations will hold for payment of the doctor's fee for care in hospital.

30% of all hospitalisations are for the group over 65. Hospitalisation may be a turning point in the lives of the elderly, with a variety of outcomes. To sketch the actual course of events one might consider an elderly patient with a common cardiovascular event such as a stroke. Since its serious character is readily recognisable on the basis of a telephoned description, the physician is likely to order the patient to the hospital. Admission will be secured, sometimes after verification of the event by an admitting physician and on presentation of a Medicare insurance card to the hospital representative in the admitting office. The deductible of $92 is payable on admission. So far as treatment is concerned, the sequences are, of course, quite standardised medically. After recovery from the acute crisis, the period of early convalescence will begin in the hospital. Physical therapy measures will generally be instituted in a variable manner, dependent to some extent on the hospital's resources and the availability of trained personnel. With many patients, such therapy often falls short of achieving full goals in ADL (Activities of Daily Living). Thus several weeks after admission, a number of possibilities loom:

1. *Home care.* If impairment is not severe and the patient has a favourable home to which he can go, discharge from the hospital may not require significant planning. The ambulance trip home will be paid for by Medicare. At home, in many but by no means all parts of the country, he can continue to receive care from a physical therapist, perhaps on a several times per week basis. He may also qualify for skilled nursing care through a certified home-health agency such as a local visiting nurse association. It is problematic whether he will be visited by his doctor at home at frequent enough intervals, though some such home visits may be made.

2. *Skilled nursing facility* (SNF). If the neurological deficits are more severe and slower to respond to treatment, transfer to an SNF may be considered desirable or necessary. A major criterion would be the need for physical therapy and presumably, other nursing needs. The transfer

may be dictated in part by social circumstances, as for example, if the patient lives alone.

Often at this point the first major bottleneck in the medical care system appears. With skilled nursing facilties fully occupied, the patient may have to wait for days or weeks for his turn from the waiting list. Prolongation of stay in the general hospital has been recognised as an unfortunate reality by Medicare and its fiscal intermediaries. They continue to reimburse the hospital at its usual daily rate, although the patient can no longer be certified as in need of such hospital care.

3. *Custodial care.* At this particular point in time with many patients, it may be clear that the patient does not need 'skilled nursing-care' in the restrictive sense defined by Medicare. His need may be for custodial care on an indeterminate basis. To receive this in a nursing-home in New York City may require an outlay of $150-250 per week and generally means an approval by local welfare authorities, since only a few can pay such amounts. This Medicaid processing may take some weeks, again with time spent in the general hospital unnecessarily. After certification by Medicaid and when a bed becomes available, the patient goes off to the nursing-home, which in fact is often the same facility which would be caring for the Medicare patient. If the disability is major and permanent, the patient may spend the rest of his life in such an institutional setting.

Similar considerations may govern the course of events after a myocardial infarction, an amputation, or any major illness. If the patient cannot be cared for at home, institutionalisation in a nursing-home or equivalent setting becomes necessary. A frequent reason for institutionalisation is the development of an organic mental syndrome. This may well lead to direct admission without intervening hospitalisation. It is of importance also to recognise that simple frailty and inability to cope with daily needs is a common cause for admission to an institution.

Transfers from one of the above settings to another are often fraught with communciation problems. The doctor who attends the patient in hospital may not be the one who sees him in a nursing-home and the reverse of this may also lead to a hiatus in care. A brief written summary giving the highlights of the patient's illness is the best that can ordinarily be expected. Occasionally it is possible to get a longer and more detailed history from the hospital in the course of one to several weeks. Communication between doctor and the nurse from the Visiting Nurse Service is also usually a brief exchange on an Inter Agency form, but occasionally via telephone. When there are different physicians in the different settings, lapses and difficulties are to be expected.

In other respects a critique of the medical care system for the elderly would take note of the deficiences which have also adversely affected the delivery of care for more youthful members of the population. All groups are similarly affected by a shortage of physicians, their poor distribution between urban and rural settings and their startling absence in the economically deprived areas of cities. In the blighted portions of USA cities, the so-called ghetto areas, few or no physicians may be available. Primary care is often delivered at an emergency room of a nearby hospital, generally for major disorders, but sometimes for trivia. Efforts to correct these deficiencies in the inner cities are still wholly inadequate. Attempted solutions have consisted of developing ambulatory care facilities at nearby hospitals and setting up of group practice units. To conserve medical manpower in these settings, emphasis has been placed on the services of paramedical workers including nurse practitioners, physician's assistants and other physician-sparing ancillary personnel.

Even in far more fortunate areas, deficiencies have progressed. Thus it has become increasingly difficult to secure a home visit from the doctor. The explanation usually given is that such a visit consumes too much of the doctor's time and that better services can be delivered if the physician is met at the emergency room of the community hospital or the patient is taken to the doctor's office. Physicians skilled in diagnosis and treatment in a home setting, or who have the backing of a Home Care Programme, are less likely to agree that every sick or febrile elderly patient needs to be moved from home to another setting in this manner. It is apparent that both medical practice considerations and Medicare/Medicaid Financing tend to promote rather than diminish institutionalisation.

NURSING-HOMES

The phenomenal development of nursing-homes is the most dramatic evidence of the growing trend towards institutionalisation of the elderly in the USA. These rapidly expanding institutional facilities have doubled in the past decade and now represent the single largest block of beds in the country. At the present time there are approximately one million such beds, a good deal more than the capacity of acute general hospitals. With the exception of a few institutions sponsored by philanthropic organisations, virtually all are under proprietary sponsorship, which is to say that, however regulated, they are run at a profit to the owners. Indeed, one rapidly expanding nationwide group of nursing-homes raised money in the late sixties by floating stock which was quoted on the New York Stock Exchange. The organisation experienced a rapid upward surge, 'a growth stock,' but finally outran itself fiscally and went into bankruptcy. Table 4.1 illustrates some aspects of sponsorship and care for these facilities in the pre- and post-Medicare period.

Table 4.1 Average monthly charge for care and percent distribution of residents in nursing-homes, by selected facility and resident characteristics: United States, 1964 and 1969. (From: *Dept. of Health, Education and Welfare, Publication 12-21,* by courtesy of Dept. of Health, Education and Welfare. The table includes only those residents who have lived in the nursing-home for at least a month and excludes life-care residents)

Selected characteristics	*1964*		*1969*	
	Average monthly charge (dollars)	*% Distribution of residents*	*Average monthly charge (dollars)*	*% Distribution of residents*
FACILITY CHARACTERISTICS				
Type of ownership				
Proprietary	205	60.2	343	69.3
Non-profit	154	24.0	306	21.3
Government	157	15.8	268	9.4
RESIDENT CHARACTERISTICS				
Level of patient care				
Intensive nursing care	224	31.0	374	32.5
Limited nursing care	199	28.7	334	41.4
Personal care	164	26.9	276	20.2
No nursing or personal care	109	13.5	216	5.9
Sex				
Male	171	35.0	315	30.9
Female	194	65.0	334	69.1
Age				
Under 65 years	155	12.0	276	11.5
65-74 years	184	18.9	324	16.8
75-84 years	191	41.7	338	39.2
85 years and over	194	27.5	338	32.5

A typical urban proprietary nursing-home runs up to 200 beds in size and is regulated with respect to its physical dimensions and other features. In New York City, the more recent buildings have 2-4 beds per room in contrast to previous homes where six or more in a room were not uncommon. Nursing-homes are subject to accreditation and inspection by various authorities. The fees charged, often paid through such authorities, result from negotiations based on a rough cost plus basis.

Originally, many nursing-homes were smaller, renovated houses and had less than savoury reputations with regard to level of care, quality of food and other services. Indeed so poor were many of them, that up until recent years, being sent to a nursing-home was regarded as an uncertain, if not abysmal end. However, standards for an 'extended care facility' now referred to as a 'skilled nursing facility', produced by the impact of Medicare, have led to considerable upgrading. As new facilities meeting the specifications for a modern, fireproof, uncrowded habitation have appeared, older inadequate facilities have been phased out. A small number of beds are occupied in some institutions by 'private patients'. They may be entitled to single room occupancy but generally pay a higher rate than that charged to governmental funding agencies.

Under Medicare the patient who has been hospitalised for three days or longer and is still in need of skilled nursing care can be transferred to a nursing-home, with Medicare reimbursement continuing for up to sixty days. However, during the first few years after Medicare went into effect, burgeoning expenditures on such nursing facilities led to a restrictive redefinition of skilled nursing care. This was a retrenchment similar to that which had occurred with the home-health services provision of Medicare, where, too, cutbacks were instituted by redefining skilled nursing. Because of this and the refusal by some authorities to pay for bills submitted, some nursing-home proprietors chose not to accept Medicare patients.

Nursing-homes have become increasingly expensive, even when the major service delivered is custodial care. Rising costs of personnel and food superimposed on rising costs of construction and financing, produced increases similar to, though less dramatic than, the huge rises in hospital care. Over the last decade patient costs in nursing-homes have risen from under $10 per day to $30 or more per day. Thus the annual bill for a patient can easily run to $10 000 or more. Very few families are in a financial position to pay out such sums, except over brief periods. As a result, virtually all the long-term patients in nursing-homes are paid for under Medicaid legislation. In essence this represents cost sharing by the Federal Government (50%), the State (25%) and the local government (25%).

At present, a *mélange* of local, state and national regulations govern the conduct of affairs in nursing-homes. These are concerned with such matters as visits by doctors, e.g. in New York City, a visit is required every thirty days. Nursing-homes are subject to inspection with regard to their hygiene, food preparation, quality of nursing and personal care delivered, with revocation of licensing a potential outcome for serious inadequacies. Although recently built homes are physically much improved for delivering nursing care, they remain remarkably unequipped for aiding the doctor in his care. Elementary procedures such as urinalysis or chest X-rays, even a haematocrit, cannot be performed on the premises. Instead, specimens are sent out to laboratories with resultant hiatuses in care. The patient who falls is sent to the emergency room of a nearby hospital for X-rays or other necessary evaluations. Notable exceptions with respect to those deficits are the non-profit nursing-homes under religious and philanthropic sponsorship. These superior homes, unfortunately in a minority, often have excellent diagnostic facilities.

The present law requires that a skilled nursing-home have a 'transfer agreement' with a nearby hospital. The essence of this is an understanding on the part of both institutions that patients may be reciprocally exchanged as indicated by medical or nursing needs. However, nursing-homes have been subject to full occupancy and have less turnover of beds than one might anticipate in a first look at their decrepit populations. This has resulted in long waits in hospital for transfer to a nursing-home, even for the patient with a priority on return to his original facility.

The salient characteristics of the population found in USA nursing-homes are variable, as one may infer from Table 4.1. There is a great range in capacity for ADL: some are ambulatory and chiefly in need of custodial care, others are limited to wheelchairs or barely get about with a walkerette and a significant number are bedridden. A recent survey of the population in one 200-bed nursing-home served by Montefiore Hospital's Home Care Department revealed the following: 53% ambulatory to some extent, 40% confused, 30% incontinent of urine, 28% wheelchair bound, 25% post stroke, 13% diabetic, 10% required feeding. The median age was 81.7 years and 80% were women (Rossman *et al.*, 1974)

Some further aspects of this sector of care and changes pre- and post-Medicare are illustrated in Table 4.1. To be noted is the fact that about one-fifth of the total population in nursing-homes are there for personal care (help with dressing, bathing, eating), not for nursing care and 5% are independent and in the institution for custodial reasons only.

A noteworthy development which is leading to further change in the composition of the nursing-home population is the transfer policy adopted by a number of states for their hospitalised mentally ill. State mental hospitals are often large institutions containing myriad elderly patients with controlled or burnt out psychoses and others chiefly with organic mental syndromes. Over the past few years, in part because

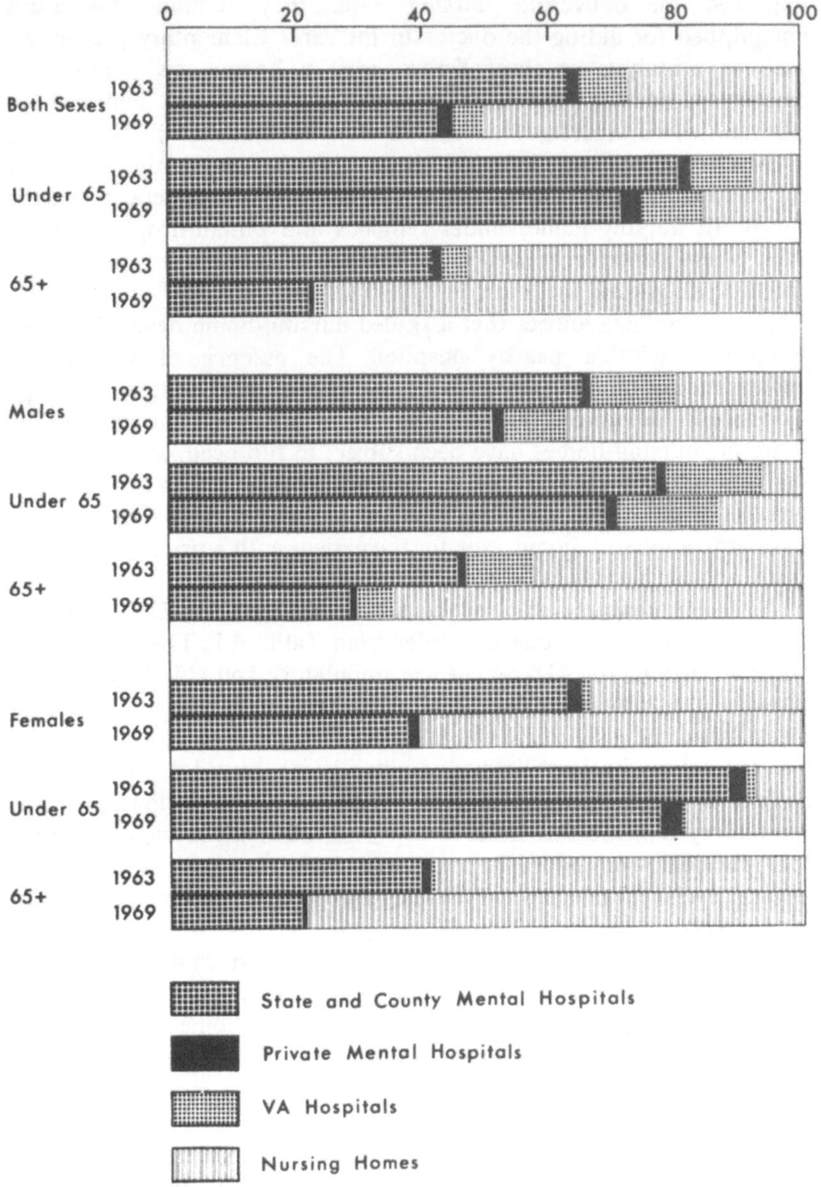

Figure 4.1 Per cent distribution of patients with mental disorders resident in selected long-term institutions by age and sex, United States: 1963 and 1969. (From, Morton, K. (October 1973). Historical tables on changes in patterns of use of psychiatric facilities. 1946-1971, by courtesy of Biometry Branch, OPPE. Nat. Inst. Mental Health)

these patients had allegedly reached a plateau and were receiving only custodial care, transfer to nursing-homes has become increasingly common. The typical nursing-home has no programming adapted to these patients and in theory is not supposed to retain patients who are a danger to themselves or to others. California has facilities called 'L' facilities, light mental facilities which are locked. Many aged patients who are mentally ill and live in California end up in an 'L' facility.

Occasionally an urgent transfer back to the hospital has become necessary because of suicidal threats or florid psychotic ideation. The graph (Figure 4.1) points up the redistribution of mentally-ill patients between hospitals and nursing-homes that occurred from 1963 to 1969, a process that has since been accelerated. Among the problem-patients thus added to the nursing-homes have been wanderers, careless smokers who start fires and irrationally aggressive or grossly paranoid individuals. Many of them have been subdued by sedation or a posey belt or jacket. Nursing-home operators point out in defence that low rates of remuneration make it impossible to hire adequate staff. Thus alternative treatment, such as one-to-one psycho-therapeutic relationships or group therapy cannot exist. Even a decade ago, before the great wave of expansion, a census had revealed the large number of psychiatrically-ill elderly in nursing-home and allied facilities. (Table 4.2).

OTHER FACILITIES FOR MENTAL ILLNESS

The most notable change in the care of mental illness has been the trend away from the state mental hospital in recent years, a trend that has been accelerating for the older age group. Traditionally, the states have been responsible for the care of mental illness requiring hospitalisation. This resulted in the building of large mental hospitals which often turned out to be grim and forbidding institutions. For example, in the State of New York, some of them ranged up to 2000 beds and though the majority of patients came from urban settings, the hospitals were mostly built out in the countryside. Shortages of psychiatrists and other skilled personnel, plus budgetary restraints, severely limited their capacity to give adequate care. There were variable, often rudimentary recreational facilities or opportunities for occupational and work therapies. Because of the very great disproportion between patient population and psychiatrists, there was virtually no psychotherapy. Introduction of the phenothiazine tranquillisers, development of psychiatric facilities within general hospitals and the above mentioned policy of discharge to nursing homes and other community facilities, has greatly reduced the number

Table 4.2 Number of residents with mental disorders and senility in nursing-homes and related facilities by age and sex, United States, May-June 1964. (From Socio-Economic Characteristics of Admissions to In-Patient Services of State and County Mental Hospitals (1971). *Department of Health, Education and Welfare, Statistics, Series A.*, No. 8, by courtesy of Dept. of Health, Education and Welfare)

	Number of residents						
	All ages	*Under 45*	*45-64*	*Total 65+*	*65-74*	*75-84*	*85+*
Both sexes							
Total, all disorders	249 159	8669	26 287	214 203	44 960	98 798	70 445
Chronic brain syndrome (CBS) with senile brain disease							
CBS with psychosis (international classification of disease -ICD - code 304)	120 974	978	1737	118 259	15 150	55 665	47 444
Senility (ICD code 794)	27 438	257	653	26 528	4311	12 703	9514
Other specified mental disorders without mention of senility (ICD codes 300-303, 305-329)	10 128	611	3777	5740	2551	2415	774
Mental or nervous trouble ill-defined (ICD codes 327, 780.7, 798.8)	90 619	6823	20 120	63 676	22 948	28 015	12 713

Note: Includes geriatric hospitals.

of admissions of the elderly to state hospitals and the duration of stay there. Nonetheless the elderly are still the largest single grouping in these institutions. Many have organic brain syndromes, others are schizophrenics who have grown old in the institutional setting.

The inevitable stigma associated with having a mental illness and especially being placed in a state hospital has been prevalent in the USA and still exists. Two categories of mentally-ill aged individuals did not end up in state institutions. One group were the wealthy who sought private psychiatric help and could afford such expenses as constant surveillance by attendants and nurses. In another category were those whose families tolerated much unusual and inappropriate behaviour without attempting to force hospitalisation. In some areas many elderly patients were maintained at home because of the community support system. The residents of a small town or farming community were often quite aware that some elderly citizens were strange. Their behaviour was taken in stride by all, with the families continuing to maintain responsibility. Needless to say, in such isolated settings, no psychiatric care was possible.

The dramatic trend in most of the state hospital systems towards returning some of their patients to the 'community' has shifted many of them virtually unsupervised into single room occupancy hotels and similar settings. This has led to many problems. At the time of this writing, for instance, the Governor of the state of California has stopped closing down parts of the hospital system because of the increasing crime through the state committed by ex state-hospital inmates. Although there are no exact figures to indicate how many of the more than 20 million persons over 65 in the USA are in need of psychiatric services, it is known that less than 3% of them have received services in psychiatric out-patient clinics. Other deficits may be traced to the widely held and inaccurate belief that elderly persons are not amenable to psychotherapy. This attitude has been changing, albeit slowly, due to the efforts of such American psychiatrists as Busse, Butler, Goldfarb, Linden, Pfeiffer and Wang, all of whom have reported positive results for psycho-therapeutic intervention.

It is well-known that there is a high incidence of withdrawal, loneliness and depression among the elderly. These are among the contributing factors to a high rate of suicide. (Table 4.3) In the USA in 1968 there were 21 281 suicides of which 5967 were over age 60. Thus 28% of the suicides were in the elderly and one may be additionally certain that the figures are gross under-reportings. It is known that the suicide prevention centres scattered throughout the United States are seldom used by the elderly. One reason may be that many old people do not have a telephone; many do not always think of turning to mental health professionals for help. The linear increase in the suicide rate with age continues to be a challenge, with the greatest population at risk being elderly white males as indicated in Table 4.3.

Table 4.3 Suicide rates in the USA for 1966 by age, sex, and colour (per 100 000). (From *Vital Statistics of the United States*, Volume II, *Mortality, Part A*, (1968) Washington, D.C.: US Public Health Service) by courtesy of US Public Health Service)

Age range	*White males*	*White females*	*Non-white males*	*Non-white females*
15-19	6.7	2.1	4.8	2.4
20-24	14.2	4.5	14.1	3.6
25-29	16.1	6.8	17.3	6.4
30-34	18.4	8.8	18.6	6.0
35-39	21.0	10.2	12.6	3.6
40-44	24.4	12.3	10.2	2.6
45-49	27.5	13.1	15.1	4.4
50-54	32.8	12.8	12.9	2.6
55-59	37.6	12.1	14.6	4.4
60-64	39.3	10.7	14.1	2.2
65-69	37.8	10.1	16.4	3.4
70-74	40.0	9.3	13.5	4.1
75-79	48.7	7.9	15.6	2.0
80-84	55.4	6.7	15.1	3.4
85-plus	59.0	4.3	23.9	3.3

Alcoholism is another major problem in the elderly. A fair number of hospitalised aged persons are diagnosed as 'chronic brain syndrome secondary to alcoholism.' Though some of these are individuals with a life-long history of consuming large amounts of alcohol, others may have adopted this method of coping in their later years. One striking finding of the study of arrests done by Epstein *et al.* (1968) was that slightly more than 80% of all arrests of persons who were 60 and older were for drunkeness.

With Federal backing, community mental health services emerged in 1963. They were required to offer a minimum of five services: In-patient care, out-patient care, partial hospitalisation, e.g. day care and twenty-four hour emergency service. A fifth component is community education and consultation services oriented towards prevention. According to the National Institute of Mental Health only 3% of the persons receiving these services were over 65 as noted above. Barriers to their use have included the stigma of mental illness, transportation problems and a lack of understanding by the generation to which the elderly belong, of the applicability of psychiatry. It is thus clear that the centres are not adequately serving the aging mentally ill. In the study by

Glasscote *et al.* (1969) some of the reasons why these centres have not decreased the admission of mentally-ill persons to state hospitals are discussed. It is well-known that the centres have difficulty in locating qualified staff to work with the mentally-ill aged. There is a lack of interest on the part of many professionals in this group and many of them have become accustomed to treating a younger population.

Since the predominant psychiatric diagnosis in the elderly requiring institutionalisation is chronic brain syndrome (Table 4.2) the thorniness of the problem is clear. Even when they are not associated with paranoid reactions and depressions, the underlying disorder still escapes reversibility. However, there may be reversible mental health problems in some brain damaged persons which are overlooked (Pollack and Goldfarb, 1961). The omnipresence of this diagnosis is indicated by one study in San Francisco where 90% of those admitted to psychiatric units of a large general hospital suffered from organic brain syndrome (Simon, 1973).

OTHER FACILITIES FOR THE AGED

In an ADL evaluation of a typical nursing-home population, a significant group can be classified as frail ambulants. This is also recognised by assigning this group to the ground floor of the institution, away from the smells of incontinence and the cries of the confused. It can be persuasively argued that this group should not be in a nursing-home at all, but in some alternative facility, in which skilled nursing care is not a necessary component. 26% of nursing-home beds in the USA are in fact occupied by a group not in need of nursing services (Table 4.1), many of whom can walk to a dining room. Transfer to a different facility might be advantageous both to patients and the governmental authorities working with increasingly strained budgets. Foster homes and institutional alternatives to nursing-homes have been variously defined in different states reflecting the broad range of patient characteristics.

Health-related facilities

At the present time in New York State, the rapid expansion of nursing-home beds seems to have come to an end. Instead health-related facilities (HRF) are being built. It is to these facilities that the less sick, ambulatory subgroup of the nursing home population will be transferred. The HRF will be geared to far simpler needs and hence should be much less costly. Patients will be ambulatory, will go to a dining room and feed themselves and be capable of taking their own medications, perhaps with some supervision. HRFs are currently being built in conjunction with standard nursing-homes. This development is envisaged as leading to tighter definitions for each category of patients and enabling ready transfers from the more skilled to the less skilled facility. In other states, homes for the aged, essentially custodial, bed and board institutions, are seen as answers to the needs of the more able subgroup currently shunted into skilled nursing-homes.

Intermediate care facilities

A further variant, the intermediate care facility (ICF) is defined as an institution to which patients with minor rather than major nursing needs may be sent. One proposal holds that for such a facility in rural areas, where a shortage of registered nurses often exists, an RN may be required only five days a week. Her essential function would be supervisory, with nursing care delivered by aides and practical nurses. In sum, geriatric population pressure is leading to alternatives to skilled nursing-homes for those with greater capability in ADL or lesser need for nursing care. There is the hope that the patients' needs will be adequately met and that costs will be significantly lowered.

Programme for the homebound

A two-year national health census (1966-1968) on illness and disability confirmed the earlier findings of Shanas *et al.* (1968) regarding the quantitative aspects of the disabled homebound. In the 65-74 age group, the figure ranged from 3.0% to 5.9% in different geographic regions. In the 75 and over group, percentages ranged from 10.3 to 17.2 with the South again heading the list. The figures for the South are higher because of the existence of an impoverished elderly black population and lessened availability of institutional facilities. According to the study, most of the necessary personal care services were delivered by relatives. Although the dimensions of the problem are now well-known, solutions have historically been entirely inadequate despite a quarter of a century's efforts, illustrated by the history of organised home care programmes.

A modern and sophisticated form of home care was launched at Montefiore Hospital in New York City in 1948. With a basic initial team of doctor, nurse and social worker, it demonstrated that a significant ungrading of services could be delivered to the home. The programme supplied equipment including hospital beds and oxygen, drugs and most important, orientation, teaching and support to the caring relatives in the home. At its maximum the team also included physiotherapists, speech therapist and occupational therapists. All members of the team met at stated conferences for patient planning and to exchange observations and data. The programme has been characterised as hospital-based, coordinated, comprehensive home care (Cherkasky *et al.*, (1961). Important categories of illness included stroke, arthritis, cancer, heart disease. Though some patients were children, a majority were over 65. The Montefiore Programme demonstrated that many patients ordinarily cared for in an institutional setting could receive an excellent quality of care in the home setting. In addition, there was documentation that such home care prevented rehospitalisation or shortened hospital stays. Although widely praised for its quality of care, its cost effectiveness and its demonstration of the values of home care, the growth of similar programmes was quite slow. A survey a decade later revealed hardly more than a hundred such comprehensive home care programmes. The failure to have a greater impact on the health care system has been ascribed to a variety of factors: difficulty in their financing, shortage of personnel, increasing specialisation of physicians and an overall doctor shortage and the growing atmosphere of negativism towards house calls to which the medical educational structure wittingly or unwittingly contributed. Many hospitals failed to concede that home care fell within their purview; others with less than full occupancy felt no pressure to generate programmes which would result in earlier discharges.

Some of the troublesome financial aspects of home care were in part resolved by the passage of Medicare Part B supplementary insurance which allowed for reimbursement of up to a hundred home visits by physicians, physical therapists and nurses and also for rental of necessary equipment. Certification standards were set up for home-health agencies, defined as agencies which were to deliver nursing care plus at least one other service. Most certified home-health agencies turned out to be pre-existent Visiting Nurse or local Health Department nursing services rather than new-formed hospital-based programmes modelled after the one at Montefiore. Recruitment of scarce personnel such as physical therapists continued to be a limiting factor as did the shortage of primary care practitioners. These limitations are to be seen in Table 4.4 which illustrates the variety of sponsorship and limitation of services.

In spite of its relatively minor role, disbursing authorities in Washington, perturbed over mounting Medicare expenditures, chose to select home care as one area for economising. This was done by issuing a restrictive definition of 'skilled nursing care'. Services which had for many years been considered appropriate for a nursing visit to a home were thereby decreed reimbursable no longer. Many home-health

Table 4.4 Number and per cent of certified home-health agencies providing selected services, by type of agency, January 1969. (From Ryder, C., Stitt, P. and Elkin, W. (1969). Home-health services—Past, present, future. *Amer. J. Pub. Health,* Vol. 59, September, by courtesy of Ames. J. Pub. Health)

		Physical therapy		*Occupational therapy*		*Speech therapy*		*Medical social service*		*Home-health aide*		*Nutrition guidance*	
Type of agency	*Number of agencies*	*Number*	*%*	*Number*	*%*	*Number*	*%*	*Number*	*%*	*Number*	*%*	*Number*	*%*
All agencies	2161*	1571	72.7	352	16.3	477	22.1	432	20.0	1042	48.2	393	18.2
Visiting Nurse Association	541	461	85.2	112	20.7	140	25.9	78	14.4	245	45.3	45	8.3
Combined government and voluntary	107	85	79.4	25	23.4	36	33.6	18	16.8	54	50.5	22	20.6
Official health	1294	830	64.1	129	10.0	193	14.9	214	16.5	589	45.5	203	15.7
Hospital based	172	154	89.5	62	36.0	82	47.7	98	57.0	1126	73.2	104	60.5
Rehabilitation facility based	12	12	100.0	11	91.7	10	83.3	7	58.3	5	41.7	3	25.0
Extended care facility based	15	12	80.0	5	33.3	7	46.7	5	33.3	11	73.3	9	60.0
Proprietary	20	17	85.0	8	40.0	9	45.0	12	60.0	12	60.0	7	35.0

Based on 2161 of the 2184 certified agencies for which data were available

Source of basic data: Social Security Administration (type of agency and services provided from application form SSA-1313)

agencies then found their routine nursing claims disallowed or not approved. As an example, consider a hemiplegic who has finished his physical therapy, but is at home with a decubitus ulcer and has a catheter. Changing dressings for the decubitus ulcer and irrigation of the catheter no longer qualified as skilled nursing care under the new restrictive interpretation. It was explained that a family member with some teaching could adequately perform these tasks. As a result, expenditures for home care under Medicare dropped in ensuing years. The $78.8 million spent in 1968 was thus lowered to $49.5 million in 1971, in contrast to the rises experienced in expenditures in the hospital and nursing home areas. There are many critics of the Medicare programme who see the failure to spend more on home care, especially supportive services, as a major weakness and over the long-term, self-defeating in keeping down the costs of care.

OTHER SIGNIFICANT TRENDS

The passage of Medicare/Medicaid legislation has produced a variety of critical reviews. Criticisms have focused on overinstitutionalisation, Medicaid inadequacies and other developments not in the best interest of the elderly. Administrators have ben appalled by rapidly mounting expenditures, far in excess of those originally contemplated. Trends and countertrends rapidly became apparent. Under the 'usual and customary fee' proviso, many physicians submitted claims which often were variably higher than those previously charged to elderly poor individuals. Because of the wide range in fees charged and some of the gross inequities in disbursements, the Medicare authorities promulgated lists of standard fees, defined as representing the usual fee charged by 75% of the practitioners in a geographic area for the procedure.

Despite some grumbling from physicians about the lowering of the allowable fee and difficulties in collecting the rest from patients, there is little doubt that USA practitioners have been made significantly richer by Medicare. More important there has been strong feeling in many quarters that for the vast sums being disbursed by Medicare, a fragmented system has been maintained, lacking comprehensiveness and coordination and with little emphasis on home care and preventive care. The consumer population has complained of rises in their monthly charges and the increase in the deductible for hospital stays. One of the government's answers to the problems of controlling fees and overdelivery of services by physicians, as well as overlong stays in institutions, has been the setting up of various review organisations. Such utilisation review groups have become increasingly important in monitoring appropriateness of care and other aspects of the quality and quantity of care.

One area of expensive and often inappropriate care has been the nursing-home. Hearings before the USA Senate have called attention to the increasing needs for community home-health services and the studious neglect of this area by Medicare (see *Home Health Services in the United States: A working paper on current status*). Various projections have indicated that a system of supportive services might conceivably care for as many as 23% of the institutionalised elderly at home or in some intermediate care facility. A good many could be shifted into an environment characterised by supervisory shared living, possibly some variant of the health related facility. In general, the USA experience validates the findings elsewhere, that the elderly present a spectrum of needs which for many reasons should not be primarily solved by institutionalisation. Anyone familiar with the possibilities of home care services in shortening hospital stays and in preventing hospitalisation will readily recognise the disproportion in the 1971 expenditures by Medicare, where $900 was spent on hospital coverage for every $1 spent on home-health services.

Transportation

Studies have shown that transportation problems are a considerable barrier confronting the elderly. One survey in New York City demonstrated that the most frequent reason for elderly persons leaving their neighbourhood was to make visits to the doctor. For the frail or handicapped, this may call for a major expenditure of strength and endurance and may even present some hazards. A few experimental projects have attempted to cope with the transportation problem. One, 'Dial-A-Ride', was a subsidised taxi-cab service which gave door-to-door transportation to the elderly on a reduced fare basis. Transportation problems will doubtless be a significant hindrance to the utilisation of congregate meal sites and day care centres.

Housing

Adequate and adaptive housing has been a significant need in many USA cities. As neighbourhoods change and decay, the elderly often are isolated in pockets of poverty. If unable to move from such areas, they find themselves confronted with increasing crime rates, the disappearance of familiar stores and even a movement away of such basic institutions as churches, banks and small hospitals. This impoverishment of the environment plus realistic considerations of personal safety have been significant in the movement of some elderly individuals into institutions. It has been widely recognised that alternative housing with supportive features for the elderly is a major unmet need. Some outstanding projects for the elderly have been built or are planned, but numerous financial and other barriers remain.

One recent solution for the more well-to-do has been newly constructed leisure villages. These have sprung up in various parts of the country, frequently in the warmer states such as Florida, Arizona and California. They vary from small enclaves to full-sized towns. Retirement villages may specify a lower age limit, but even in the absence of such a limit, are overwhelmingly composed of retirees 60 and older. Although the initial population may be ambulatory and in good health, with the passage of the years and the inevitable onslaught of disabilities, increasing needs for medical and hospital care arise. These may not be met satisfactorily, especially for home care. Some of the other problems associated with communities composed of the elderly are well-known. Segregation by age eventually becomes a depressive criterion to which the elderly themselves may object.

Nutrition

A number of surveys have demonstrated that because of poverty, isolation, weakness or apathy, the elderly suffer from malnutrition in significant numbers. One major recommendation of the 1971 White House Conference on Aging called for allocation of funds for nutritional programmes; this is to be translated into action in 1974. Under the law the states will receive funds in proportion to the number of elderly residing within them. Grants will be given to establish congregate meal sites. These are to serve at least a hundred meals per day, five days a week. Eligible individuals will be those 60 and over. There are provisions for home-delivered meals in coordination with the congregate meal site, if this be deemed necessary to serve the bedridden or homebound. The law also requires that supporting social services be made available. With an appropriation for the year of approximately $100 million it is estimated that approximately 250 000 persons 60 and over may be able to take part in the programme. However, attention must be called to the fact that there are almost 30 million individuals in this age category, with 5 million living in poverty. Also, the programme seems applicable chiefly to the urban poor and not to those in rural areas.

Other developments

In 1972, another programme designed to meet the needs of the homebound was launched, also at Montefiore Hospital. Termed the After Care Programme (ACP), this demonstration project showed that many of the patients typical of a Home Care Programme could be brought into a designated area of the hospital, using vans for wheelchair-bound patients. A common denominator for a group might be a need for physical therapy, as for example, arthritis or hemiplegia. A typical group consisted of six patients who received physical, occupational, recreational and other therapies, plus access to doctor, nurse and social worker in the course of a three-hour stay. Advantages for ACP included more efficient use of personnel, increased range of services to patients and, interestingly enough, patient preference over traditional home care. The impact of this demonstration remains to be seen, but it is clearly a viable alternative to home care and possesses certain built-in advantages (Rossman, 1974).

Geriatric day care hospitals are virtually non-existent in the USA. Some have come and gone over the years, disappearing in part because of unsustained financial support. Their value and importance in England have been clearly documented by Brocklehurst (1970). There has been a recent rekindling of interest in the applicability of day hospitals with one currently in operation in a community building on the Montefiore Hospital grounds. As an additional straw in the wind, New York State authorities have proposed that health-related facilities offer day care as an appropriate added service. If the exploration of alternatives to institutionalisation continues full force, day care will doubtless assume increased importance.

Geriatric nurse practitioner

Geriatrics is not a recognised subspecialty in the USA and the educational structure (medical school plus teaching hospital) has largely neglected it. There is thus an acute shortage of geriatricians. There have been a number of attempts to rectify this shortage. Programmes are now beginning to educate nurses for an expanded role as geriatric nurse practitioners. Nurse practitioners have been developed in paediatrics, maternal and child health, and in the adult family health sector. A joint practice committee of doctors from the AMA and nurses from the ANA was formed in 1973 and met to delineate the roles of geriatric nurse practitioner who will be a registered nurse with special schooling and will be able to work collaboratively with physicians and others in meeting health needs of geriatric patients. In addition, she will be able to perform other functions such as obtaining a comprehensive health history and performing a physical examination, prescribing selected medications according to standard orders, making decisions prospectively and cooperatively with the doctor, in addition to decisions involving the level of traditional nursing judgements and teaching and counselling patients and family regarding aging processes in health and illness.

Senior centres

These are chiefly recreational or get-together places for older people, sponsored by community agencies or housing authorities. A few have social services, informational programmes, or are involved in meal preparation and health counselling. It is anticipated that many more will be involved in projected meal programmes and that the centres could serve as a base for a variety of activities. There are more than ninety in New York City alone, with another sixty planned and in 1972 the total for the United States was around 1200.

SUMMARY

The care system for the elderly in the USA has only recently emerged from a wasteland of neglect which was littered with a hodge-podge of random solutions. Medicare insurance, a major turning point, focuses mainly on hospitalisation and ambulatory care. Medicaid's added contribution consists of a heavy accent on nursing-home solutions. For multiple reasons, home care services have been honoured more in the breach than the observance despite excellent demonstrations of their usefulness. Thus there are still many inadequacies and strains when prolonged illness or chronic disability are present. It seems inevitable that a broader range of supportive services and planning will have to emerge, a development that has been made the more necessary by the continuing existence of financial hardships for the insured elderly poor. Current trends suggest that among new directions will be congregate living and dining sites, geriatric centres for ambulatory care and intermediate facilities of various grades that will correspond to the spectrum of needs. Shortages of skilled personnel and the staggering cost of the present system will accelerate the search for further non-institutional solutions.

References

Brocklehurst, J. C. (1970). *The Geriatric Day Hospital,* 100 (King Edwards Hospital Fund for London)

Cherkasky, M., Rossman, I. and Rogatz, P. (1961). *Guide to Organized Home Care,* 34 (Chicago: Hospital Research Educational Trust)

Epstein, L. J., Mills, C. and Simon, A. (1968). *The Elderly Offender: I. The Elderly Alcoholic: The Jail is a Substitute for Hospitalisation*

(Read at the Annual Meeting of the Gerontological Society. Denver, Colorado. October 31-November 2)

Glasscote, P. M., Sussex, J. N., Cumming, E. and Smith, L. H. (1969). *The Community Mental Health Center: An Interim Appraisal* (Washington, D.C.: The Joint Information Services at the Psychiatric Association and the National Association for Mental Health)

Home Health Services in the United States: A working Paper on Current Status. Special Committee on Aging. U.S. Senate Washington, D.C.: (U.S. Government Printing Office Publication 5270-0874)

Pollack, M. and Goldfarb, A. I. (1961). Factors related to individual differences in the mental health of institutionalized aged. In: *Psychopathology of Aging,* 104-113 (P. H. Moch and J. Zubin, editors) (New York: Grure and Stratton, Inc.)

Rossman, I. (1974). The after care project: A viable alternative to home care. *Medical Care,* **12,** 534-540

Rossman, I., Rodstein, M. and Bornstein, A. (1974). Undiagnosed diseases in an aging population. Pulmonary embolism and bronchopneumonia. *Arch. Int. Med.,* **133,** 366-369

Shanas, E. (1962). *The Health of Older People. A Social Survey,* 250 (Harvard University Press)

Shanas, E., Townsend, P., Wedderburn, D., Friis, H., Milhoj, P. and Stenhouwer, J. (1968). *Old People in Three Industrial Societies* (New York: Atherton Press)

Simon, A. (1973). The psychology of aging In: *Aging: Prospects and Issues* (R. H. Davis, editor) (Ethel Percy Andrus Gerontology Center, University of Southern California, Los Angeles, California)

Suggested reading

Atchley, R. C. (1972). Health. In: *The Social Forces in Later Life* (Belmont, California: Wadsworth Publishing Company) (Has excellent bibliography with this chapter)

Burnside, I. M. (ed.) (1973). *Psychosocial Nursing Care of the Aged* (New York: McGraw Hill Book Company) (Has one section devoted to group work by nurses)

Busse, E. W. and Pfeiffer, E. (1973). *Mental Illness in Later Life* (Washington, D.C.: American Psychiatric Association)

Butler, R. N. and Lewis, M. I. (1973). *Aging and Mental Health* (St. Louis: C. V. Mosby Co.)

Jaeger, D. and Simmons, L. W. (1970). *The Aged Ill* (New York: Appleton-Century-Crofts)

Stotsky, B. A. (1968). *The Elderly Patient* (New York: Grune and Stratton, Inc.)

Symposium (1973). Problems of Older people: Forced idleness, impoverishment, ill health, isolation. 1973 Health Conference. The New York Academy of Medicine. *Bull. N. Y. Acad. Med.,* December 1973 Volume 49, No. 12

CHAPTER FIVE

Sweden

Alvar Svanborg

HISTORY OF MEDICAL CARE FOR OLD PEOPLE

Organised care of the debilitated and the chronically ill was present in the Swedish community as early as the Middle Ages. Institutions were organised and, since these included the care of patients with infectious diseases, were, in most cases, built beyond city or town limits. It was tried, not infrequently, to make them into self-supporting units—large estates with their own agriculture, forestry, hunting, etc.

The first hospital for the acutely ill was founded at the end of the 17th century and was primarily intended for the care of miners, injured in the course of their work. During the 18th century acute hospitals were built, for example in Uppsala and Stockholm which, while intended for the acute medical care of patients, also had the added function of being teaching institutions. Shortly afterwards, however, the population began to appreciate the need for acute hospitals and in the 1760s units, under the guidance of the county governor, were organised in each county. The initial conditions under which these hospitals were established and controlled were laid down in a royal decree in 1817. This was followed by instructions for community epidemic hospitals in 1875 (directions for the care of cholera patients had, however, already been drawn-up earlier) and for tuberculosis institutions in 1915. In 1928 the County Council was bound by law for the first time in history to provide medical care under the conditions of the Hospital Act. It should, however, be stressed that this Act did not concern the chronically sick and convalescents. This despite the fact that there had already, for many centuries, existed institutions in which had been organised medical units on a far greater scale than those found in hospitals treating the acutely ill. Within these medical units for the chronically ill lived also invalids, those debilitated by age and the poorest in the community who, for some reason, were incapable of caring for themselves. Consequently, the mentally ill, those with tuberculosis, etc. were treated here also. A reorganisation of the mental health care began in the middle of the 19th Century in Sweden. Hospital property, at that time owned by the authorities dealing with chronically-ill patients, was sold. The influx of economic resources was taken over by the authorities in charge of the so-called Poor Aid ostensibly to assume control over the care of the chronic physically-ill patients. However, these resources were spread over both chronic and acute patients, both in the physical and mental spheres.

It was only in 1951 that the care of chronic physically-ill patients was put on an equal legal status with that of the other physically-ill patients. The plans then in existence anticipated that the community should build special units for the relatively healthy elderly members of society, i.e. old-age homes. If they became ill they should be cared for in another type of hospital, i.e. if acutely ill in an acute hospital, but in other cases in a general ward set aside for the chronically ill, or in a special home intended for the sick and, therefore, generally better equipped medically than the old-age homes. The acute medical specialties, in particular internal medicine, had earlier to a certain extent concentrated the chronically ill to special wards within the general hospital. The Hospital Act was changed in 1959 making it possible to organise special units with their own consultants for long-term care, within the framework of the general hospital.

The need for a separate specialty dealing with the care of the chronically ill and geriatric patients had been discussed very keenly, mainly by doctors and politicians, in the years following the 1959 Act. The majority were apparently in agreement that such a need existed. The problem then remained of what this special branch should be called. Some tried to introduce the term 'geriatrics', since this specialty was already organised in certain countries, e.g. in England. The main reason for not accepting this terminology seems to have been the fear, on the part of doctors and politicians alike, that hospitals would be organised in such a way that admission would be dependent not on the need for care, but on patient age. It was mainly for this reason that the specialty came to be called *long-term care medicine* when it was officially recognised in 1969.

As yet no division of long-term care medicine into subspecialties has occurred. In certain centres in Sweden special psycho-geriatricians are employed, i.e. psychiatrists with a certain amount of specialisation in long-term medicine and with a primary interest in patients with senile dementia.

Specialising in long-term medicine entails two years internal medicine, two years long-term medicine and six months psychiatry. During these four and a half years the aspirant specialist must have attended six courses, each lasting one week and finishing with a proficiency test. This postgraduate education is, in principle, the same as that within other medical specialities. Somatic long-term care is managed parallel with other medical care in Sweden.

Thus, quantitatively long-term medicine has predominated in Sweden through all the centuries up to the 20th Century. With the increase in

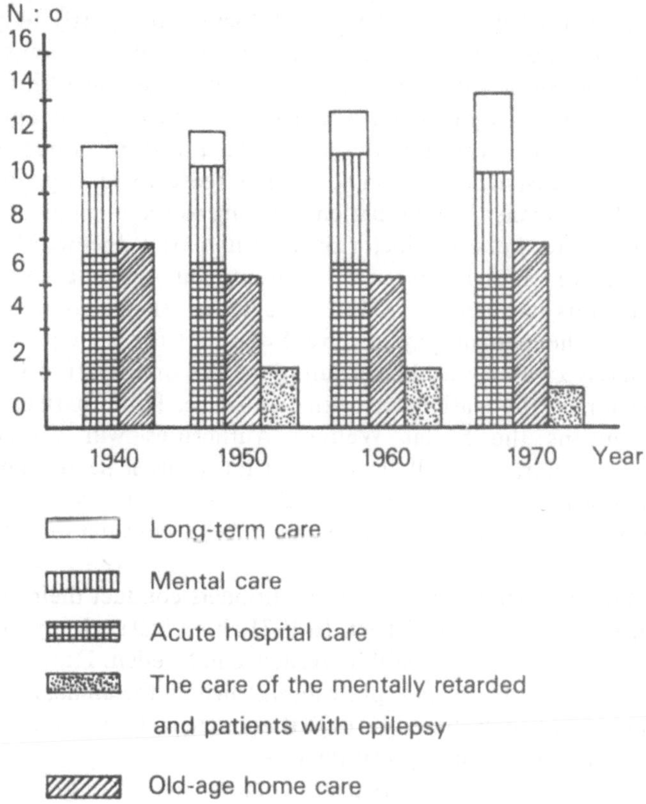

Figure 5.1 Number of beds per 1000 inhabitants in 1940-1970. From the Swedish National Board of Health and Social Welfare: "Långtidsvårdens läge", 1974. AB Allmänna Förlaget. Vällingby, Sweden.

knowledge and technical resources the main concentration of effort during the 20th Century has been focused on acute medical care and the care of chronically sick and debilitated has taken a second place. During the last decades, however, a new trend has developed in this respect and the Swedish community is beginning to show more concern for long-term care (Figure 5.1)

PRESENT SITUATION

Primary care

Public health is organised, to all intents and purposes, separately from medical care; dental care is also separate.

The primary care of ambulatory patients is carried out partly by officially appointed district and hospital doctors and partly by private general practitioners and specialists. The care of out-patients outside the hospital in the country districts has from as early as the 17th Century been taken care of by the state, which for this purpose has appointed district doctors. The communities have under certain circumstances, appointed town district doctors in addition to those doctors appointed by the state. This means that the patient wishing to see a doctor is always able to visit a rural district doctor or a town district doctor. Moreover, this category of physician is on duty twenty-four hours a day. These district doctors are paid a full salary by the community. At the moment the patient pays twelve Swedish Crowns, equivalent to approximately £1 or $3, at the consultation. The main part of the fee is then paid for by the National Health Insurance. If the patient has no financial means the Social Welfare Authorities will compensate. Necessary transportation will also be paid for, at least partly. This is of special importance in thinly populated areas (which are common in Sweden), where the doctor's surgery may be a considerable distance away.

Many of these officially appointed practitioners conduct their practices in their own surgeries in the district. In 1971 about 550 such surgeries run by doctors on their own were still in existence in Sweden. During the last decade this number has been rapidly diminished by the amalgamation of several doctors into polyclinics. In 1971 there were sixty-five clinics run by three doctors and 125 run by two doctors.

The officially appointed district doctors account for 25% of ambulatory medical care. During the last decades out-patient care has, to an ever-increasing extent, been concentrated in hospitals and it is estimated that about 50% of medical consultations (excluding X-ray and laboratory investigations) now take place in Swedish hospitals. There are about 1500 doctors employed for out-patient care alone by the community, as opposed to 6500 doctors employed for both in-patient and out-patient care in hospitals. In addition there is a certain number of private practitioners concerning themselves with out-patient work in the large centres and these account for about 25% of all out-patient care in Sweden.

The out-patient curve shows the lowest demand in the ages between 5 and 15 years and maximum demand between 55 and 67 years (Figure 5.2).

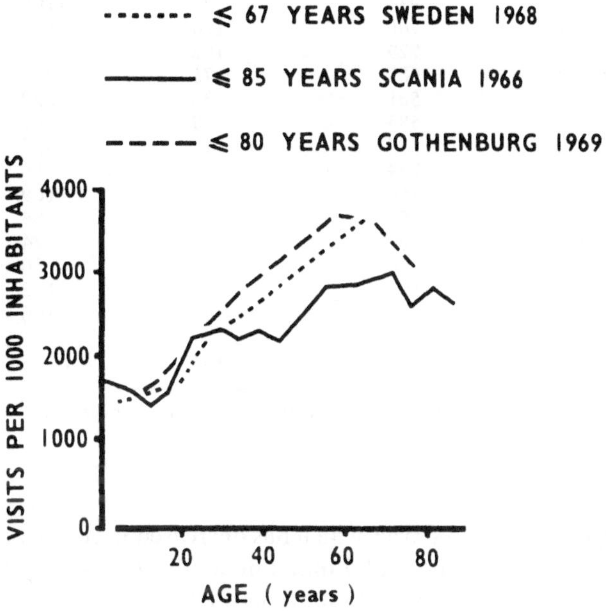

Figure 5.2 Number of out-patient visits per 1000 inhabitants annually. The three curves showing the situation in total Sweden 1968, Scania 1966 and Gothenburg 1969, resp. From the Swedish National Board of Health and Social Welfare: 'Hälso-och sjukvård inför 80-talet', 1973. Stockholm, Sweden.

The decrease in demand after 67 years of age may, to a certain extent, be explained by a greater proportion of the population in the later age group requiring medical care as in-patients. It is, naturally, always interesting to know the reasons for out-patient' consultations. A detailed description has been made recently, based on an investigation carried out in one of the large cities in Sweden, i.e. Gothenburg (Table 5.1).

Table 5.1 Analysis of out-patient consultations in Gothenburg

Diseases	*Visits by appointment to out-patient clinics*	*Visits without appointment to clinics + home visits*	*Total*	*%*
Respiratory	1989	266	2255	14
Muscle, joint, ligaments etc.	1745	85	1830	11
Psychiatric	1520	201	1721	11
Accidents	1045	502	1547	10
Circulatory	1334	117	1451	9
Urogenital	1109	164	1273	8
Digestive	934	174	1108	7
Ear, nose and throat	706	164	870	5
Skin	729	102	831	5
Infectious Diseases	583	175	758	5
Eye	561	38	599	4
Neoplastic	583	9	592	4
Endocrine	375	17	392	2
Neurological	234	46	280	2
Haematological	164	5	169	1
Obstetrical	51	33	84	0
Congenital defects	67	7	74	0
Speech defects	30	–	30	0
Diagnosis uncertain	93	19	112	0
Unspecified	66	40	106	0
Total	13 924	2164	16 088	100

From "Oppen sjukvärd i Göteborg 1969". SPRI rapport 1/1972, page 29, by Margareta Härnqvist and Nalle Lindholm.

Home medical care is a service which has decreased in the last decades. In the study by Härnquist and Lindholm in the city of Gothenburg (1969-1970) only 2% of the consultations took place in the patient's home. Doctors in out-patient care usually work in their surgeries and home-visits are reserved mainly for the acutely ill, or for recurrences of acute illness in the chronically sick or handicapped patients. Possibilities for continuous medical care by the doctor for the chronically ill and those debilitated by age have been far from ideal. This may also explain the reduction of out-patient care demand, as shown by official statistics, in the higher age-group. It is, moreover, unusual to find a general practitioner's surgery or a general out-patient clinic sufficiently well equipped to undertake the long and detailed examination required for the severely handicapped. The main alternative in these cases has therefore been in-patient care. Unfortunately, however, these cases usually have the lowest priority on waiting lists for hospital admission.

They, therefore, accumulate on these waiting lists unexamined and untreated.

There is, however, without a doubt a great latent need for care, and investment in out-patient care for the elderly could obviate or, at least, pospone the need for in-patient care. An examination of the demand for in-patient care shows an increasingly steep curve with increase in age. Results of population studies indicate that this graph might be dextroposed by enlarged efforts for the elderly in out-patient care.

Home care is organised partly by the Health Authorities, involving district doctors and nurses and partly by the Social Welfare personnel, many of whom have some medical education, e.g. that of a registered nurse. The basic intention is that the Health Authorities shall handle all medical activities within home care. However, even the Social Welfare home care organisation has to be responsible for medical decisions and support actions, due to shortage of medical personnel.

Physicians are engaged within the administration of the Social Welfare of the communities. These organisational tasks are to an ever-increasing extent being given to long-term care hospital doctors. It is rather unusual for the long-term specialist to undertake home visits. Instead the patient or his relatives or the Social Welfare workers call for the district doctors or private practitioners. Unfortunately their activities are dominated by consultations at the office and home calls get secondary priority as a rule.

In spite of the fact that the number of physicians per 1000 inhabitants (1.5 pro mille as of 1st January 1973) is not particularly low from an international point of view, the main part of out-patient care is concentrated on acute illness and on care of other groups of patients with relatively well-defined diseases and proportionately less on the care of severely disabled elderly patients.

There are now in Sweden plans to break this trend by strengthening the family doctor function and by enlarging the possibility offering home care. For this purpose there will be a more extended postgraduate training for 'specialists' in general medicine.

Contributions to out-patient care in hospitals by long-term medicine

Many, if not most, of the patients newly admitted to long-term medical units by district doctors or private practitioners are, even by the time they are put on the waiting list too ill or handicapped to be accepted as out-patients in either general practice or acute out-patient departments in hospital. In certain hospitals an attempt has been made to organise out-patient departments specially equipped for the examination and treatment of patients who are severely handicapped or debilitated by age. Such a clinic has, for example, been in existence in Vasa Hospital in Gothenburg since 1969. Adequate space and many personnel are required in such a unit. The entire long-term medical team is involved in this out-patient scheme, i.e. apart from doctors and nurses and orderlies, there must also be available physiotherapists, occupational therapists, etc. The opportunities offered by such an out-patient department can also be used by consultants in other specialities, e.g. psychiatrists, general surgeons, orthopaedic surgeons and oncologist to everyone's mutual advantage.

In acute out-patient departments there is usually a wait of many hours for non-acute patients and the investigation is divided between several consultations. A return visit is necessary for routine investigations, e.g. X-rays. The acute cases take priority. In long-term medical out-patient departments facilities are made available for immediate investigation, if possible, as the patients constitute, in the majority of cases, a transport problem.

Long-term medical patients' needs vary, over a period of time, between in-patient, day, home and out-patient care. Experience has shown that families and auxiliary workers are more willing to care for an elderly or disabled patient at home if they can rely on continuous contact with a medical team ready, if necessary, to provide the eventual care needed by the patient. This need is supplied by this special type of out-patient department and, so far, experience has shown a very hopeful result. In 1973 11 283 out-patient consultations were registered in the long-term clinics in Gothenburg. A considerable expansion of out-patient resources is, thus, an essential complement to the ever-increasingly hard-pressed long-term medical care.

Hospital care

Private hospitals are very unusual in Sweden. Almost all hospitals are run by the communities, one by the Government.

In-patient somatic long-term care is at present given in:

1. *Long-term clinics.* Many of these clinics (wards) are situated in the same hospital as the acute medical specialities. Several are, however, geographically separated and have, therefore, separate diagnostic and therapeutic resources. The Swedish long-term clinics have, in general, good resources for medical and social rehabilitation. Within the clinics, units for day care are very common and are used not only to lighten the in-patient care load but also for diagnostic and therapeutic purposes.

These clinics have also, naturally, responsibility for the training of medical personnel in the field of long-term care. The need for specialists in long- term medicine within hospital areas has become increasingly obvious and has been emphasised by the national authorities in their plans for further development of the hospital organisation. In some hospitals the main resources for medical rehabilitation are concentrated in the long-term clinics. There are in larger hospitals special clinics for medical rehabilitation, which is a recognised speciality in Sweden. Their responsibility is directed mainly to occupational training, rehabilitation of patients with neurological diseases and post-traumatic conditions. These clinics are also responsible for the principle part of the basic education of physiotherapists and occupational therapists.

2. *Nursing-homes for somatic long-term patients.* There are three different categories of nursing-homes:

(a) In a few hospital districts there are so-called central nursing-homes headed by long-term specialists, which have relatively good resources for simple rehabilitation by means of assistance supplementary to the patients' own efforts. In certain areas, e.g. Greater-Stockholm, polyclinics organised by the community are attached to these homes. The 'homes' are run by long-term specialists and the polyclinics have full-time services of consultants in several specialties, e.g. internal medicine, surgery, psychiatry, etc. These homes have access to the resources provided by the polyclinics.

(b) There are also other nursing-homes, usually geographically separated from the general hospitals in certain towns. Even these nursing homes have certain possibilities for medical rehabilitation. Usually, but not always, these nursing-homes are coordinated with the long-term clinics in hospitals or the central nursing-homes.

In both these above-named categories, central nursing-homes and nursing-homes, the word 'home' does not cover adequately the service provided by these institutions as they have responsibility for patients needing medical care, physiotherapy and occupational therapy, but not needing the diagnostic and therapeutic resources found in acute hospitals. For normal ward activities these 'homes' function in the same manner as general hospitals.

(c) In the rural districts there are also peripheral nursing-homes usually administered by the local district medical officer. These homes have, in general, limited possibilities for rehabilitation and have mainly the function of patient care by nurses. These homes are mostly intended for patients whose condition is stationary and who do not require constant medical care. These homes, moreover, have a more homely atmosphere.

3. *Special medical care units in old-age homes.* There is a bed-shortage

in long-term clinics and nursing-homes and, unfortunately, certain elderly patients have to be cared for here, despite the lack of constant medical surveillance.

4. To a small extent also in wards for somatic long-term patients in general hospitals, administered by specialties other than long-term care medicine.

5. *Acute clinics in hospitals.* Due to the shortage of beds in long-term clinics and nursing-homes many long-term cases are also treated in the acute wards in hospitals.

6. Sweden also has, albeit to a less extent, private nursing-homes having resources comparable with those of the peripheral nursing-homes.

The population of Sweden in January 1972 was 8 115 426. At that time there were a total number of 34 054 beds for long-term somatic patients together with 2114 beds in private nursing-homes (divided amongst 61 homes). The 34 054 beds included 6264 in long-term clinics (distributed over 59 units,) 16 608 in central nursing-homes (distributed over 115 units), and 11 182 in peripheral nursing-homes (distributed over 226 units) (Table 5.2). At the same time, the number of ward places in old

Table 5.2 Total resources for long term physically ill patients, Sweden, 1972

(1)	Long term clinics	6264
(2 a, b)	Central nursing homes	16 608
(2 c)	Peripheral nursing homes	11 182
	Total long term hospital beds for physical illness	34 054
(3)	Wards in old people's homes	58 407
(6)	Private nursing homes	2114
	Total	128 629
	Total population	8 115 426 (1.1 million aged 65+)

Number in brackets refer to text

people's homes was 58 407. This figure includes those relatively few elderly patients cared for in the special medical units (1486 beds in 38 units) of the old people's homes (see under 3 above).

While the population of Sweden in 1971 was 8.1 million, the calculated population in 1990 will be 8.4 million. This means an absolute increase of 310 000 and a relative increase of 3.8%. During the same period the size of the 65+ group was 1.1 million and 1.4 million, respectively, which means an absolute increase of 300 000 and a relative increase of 26.5%. In fact, out of the calculated total increase of 310 640 no less than 301 498 belong to the 65+ group, i.e. about 97%.

The calculated size and age distribution of the population 65 years and older between the years of 1970 and 2000 is seen in Figure 5.3. Up to 1990 there is an absolute increase and after 1990 the figures seem to be stationary or decrease slightly.

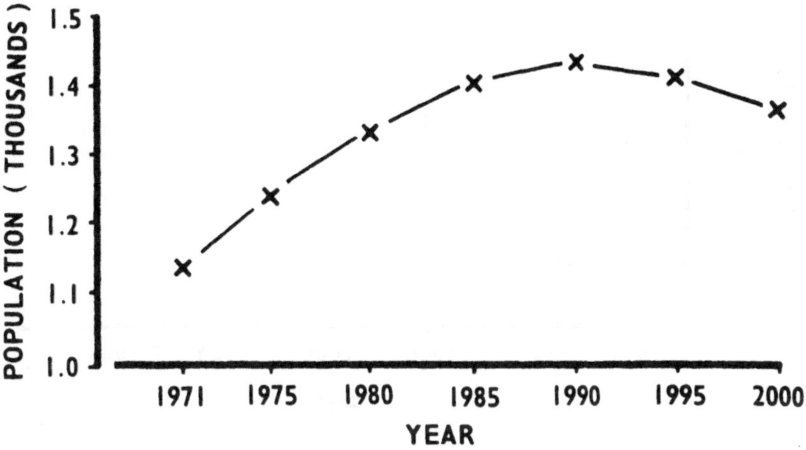

Figure 5.3 Calculated population in Sweden (immigration = 0) 65 years and older.

The calculated size of the groups of advanced age is seen in Figure 5.4, showing that the absolute increase in individuals aged 80+ will accelerate and that this increase will continue up to the 21st century, i.e. the age group requiring more constant medical care than any other group will increase dramatically and that this increase will continue during the whole century. In Figure 5.5 the accumulated relative increase of these groups is illustrated.

At the beginning of January 1972 the number of beds available for general medical somatic patients in the 70+ age group was 4.6 per 100 inhabitants of this age group. This applies generally in Sweden. However, this figure varies in practice in different circumstances, e.g. the need is greater in large towns. In an investigation carried out earlier by the authorities into the demand for hospital beds, the long-term medical requirement was estimated at being 5.5 beds per 100 inhabitants in the 70+ age group. Experience, however, has shown this to be unrealistic

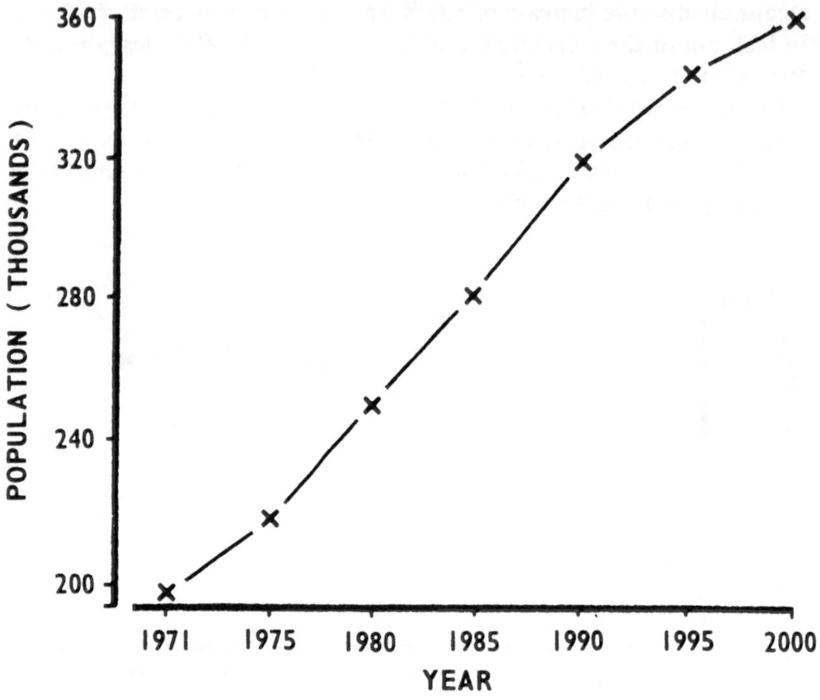

Figure 5.4 Calculated population in Sweden (immigration = 0) 80 years and older.

and the requirements, at least in the larger towns, to be appreciably larger. In these areas one can reckon with a need for 8-9 beds per 100 inhabitants in the 70+ age group.

However, a recent population study in Gothenburg indicates that the 70+ age group is relatively healthy and the need for institutional care shows in actual fact a dramatic acceleration at first in the higher age groups. This age shift has not been taken into consideration in the statistical planning of care for the elderly, which is still incorrectly calculated along a line based on the steepness of the 65+ or 70+ age group, instead of along the line which shows the change of the average care consumer in the higher age groups, i.e. those with a definitely higher need of medical care than the younger adult ages (Figures 5.3, 5.4 and 5.5). In addition to the calculated need for the high age groups, as mentioned above, must be included the need for beds for those patients with organic mental conditions such as senile dementia, arterio-sclerotic dementia, alcoholic dementia and cerebral trauma. The frequency of these conditions in the population, both in urban and rural districts, has

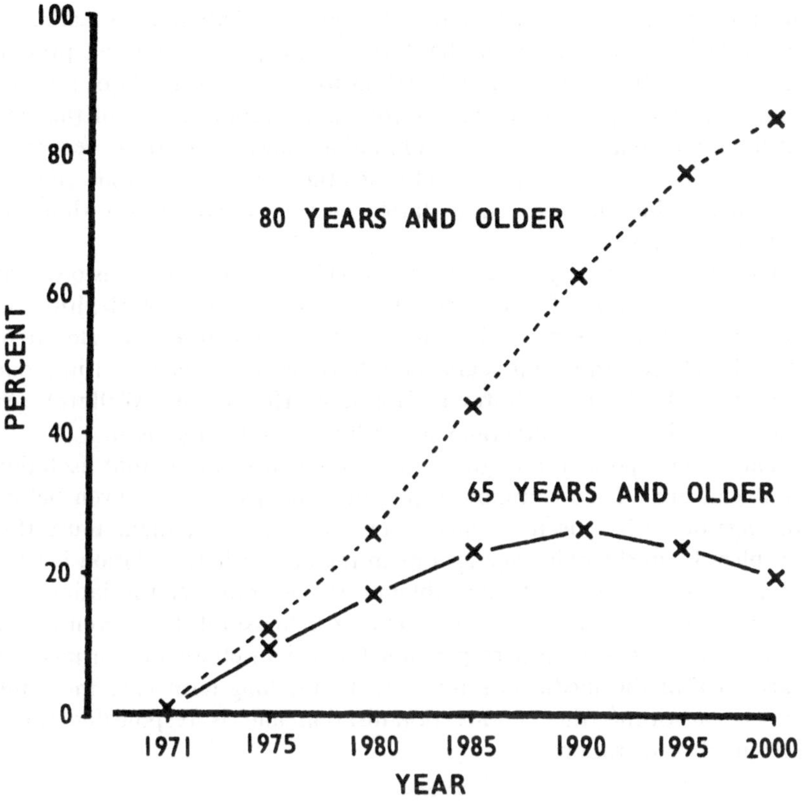

Figure 5.5 Calculated population in Sweden (immigration = 0). Cumulative relative increase in people, 80 years and older and 65 years and older, respectively.

been the subject of investigation and shows a 2% frequency in the 8th age decade and a 4-5% frequency in the 9th decade. To this figure must be added the number of those patients less demented but still, in many cases, in need of institutional care. Figures here vary but a realistic average figure seems to be 2-4% of the population in the 70+ age group. It has become traditional that patients who are agitated, disturbing to other people, or confused to such an extent that they require in-patient care, be considered as belonging to the psychiatric field. Conversely, patients in whom the somatic illness dominates are cared for mainly in somatic long-term clinics and, to a minor extent, in acute clinics. The remaining cases of dementia fall into no special category and suffer from the fact that no specialty will take the responsibility for them. These patients have been cared for, to an ever-increasing extent, either at home or in old people's homes. One may hopefully anticipate the creation of ward facilities for them in the future. The plans being at present discussed by the central administration follow the principle of somatic long-term care speciality assuming the major responsibility for the care of the senile demented, with the exception, however, of those requiring psychiatrically trained personnel and the resources found only in psychiatric institutions. These latter cases will still fall within the psychiatric sphere.

The central authority was in the past divided into two subdivisions, one having responsibility for medical care: (National Board of Health) and the other having responsibility for social welfare (National Board of Social Welfare). In recent years these have been amalgamated into one central authority (The National Board of Health and Welfare). At the county level these functions are still separately organised.

The recent population study in Gothenburg shows that isolation problems are all too common, especially amongst women, even before the age of 70 has been reached. How much greater, then, must this problem be in the older age groups in the cities where isolation is even more common? The medical problems arising from social isolation and inactivity have been focused and the aim is to establish an even closer cooperation between those responsible for social welfare and for medical care. Within the medical sector it is mainly long-term care medicine which constitutes the contact organisation and is responsible for a system of cooperation.

PROPOSED DEVELOPMENTS

A considerable expansion of somatic and mental long-term care is being planned in Sweden together with a certain decrease in the number of beds at present available to the acute medical specialties. To coincide with this, efforts are to be made to strengthen the special resources available for the care in the home of the chronically ill and those debilitated by age. An important step in achieving this aim is broadening the further education of the general practitioner. Three years' postgraduate study, both in organised courses and work within certain specialties in hospitals, will be required for full registration as a general practitioner. The efficiency of general practitioners' surgeries is also to be increased, partly by the formation of polyclinics and partly by the availability of additional help by for example nurses, physiotherapists, occupational therapists, social workers, dieticians, etc. It is also intended to increase subsidies for preventive and prophylactic medical care, not least for the most elderly in the community. An important aim is to decrease the risk inherent in physical inactivity and social and mental isolation. This aim can only be achieved after a thorough investigation into the present living conditions for the elderly in the community. It is not known whether these comprehensive health controls and population studies will be performed by representatives of the medical specialty long-term care or by general practitioners, guided by these specialists. According to the author of this chapter the population studies performed up to now speak in favour of the fact that such population studies should be based on the resources which today are available only in the long-term care departments.

The curriculum followed by medical students does not include instruction in long-term medicine/geriatrics. However, some students do have a certain amount of contact with long-term medical care. In certain university hospitals in Sweden, e.g. Gothenburg, a three-month preliminary course dealing with basic ward principles (including nursing techniques) and clinical techniques introduces the student to clinical medicine. This course is called Propedeutical Medicine and is, in certain hospitals, provided within the framework of the long-term care wards. This has proved to be ideal as long-term wards offer great experience in the subjects dealt with in these courses. This, however, cannot be considered as specialist training in long-term medicine as the students, at that stage, have not enough experience to appreciate the special problems encountered in the care of aging patients. It is essential, therefore, that a further period of training in long-term medicine, preferably towards the end of the under-graduate period, be introduced.

As yet there is only one professorial post in geriatrics. This is in Uppsala and at present fulfills a mainly theoretical function with medical research and is not directly concerned with those problems with which the specialty of long-term medicine is concerned. It is clear that university resources, must be strengthened not only for further education in long-term medicine/geriatrics, but also for research and medical evolution projects. Definite plans for such a development, however, have not been formulated.

CHAPTER SIX

The Union of the Soviet Socialist Republics

R G Revutskaya

INTRODUCTION

Health preservation of older age-groups of the population has great social and economic implications. It relates closely on the one hand to the engagement of older people in production and social activity: on the other hand, it relates to state expenditure on public health and social welfare as well as time expenditure of family members, nurses and of those who are ill and incapacitated.

To this end, in the USSR vast prophylactic and therapeutic measures have been developed arising from the present state of medical practice, mass physical culture and sanitation provision. These prophylactic-therapeutic and sanitary measures are designed to allow older people wherever possible to remain in their normal environment, to prolong their working period and to preserve mobility and the ability for self-service. A good psychic state keeps up their full social competence.

Because medical aid in the Soviet Union is public and free of charge (there arc 109.7 beds and 27.4 physicians per 10 000 people (Loginova *et al.*, 1968)) older people enjoy the rights both to in-patient and out-patient medical care and also a doctor's home visiting service (which is very important at this age). Many patients with cardiovascular and gastro-intestinal diseases are followed-up at special health centres and dispensaries.

Medical science has now accumulated significant research and practical experience in the treatment of aged patients, allowing the separation of *geriatrics* (the science of disease in old age) into an individual field. This in its turn makes it possible for physicians to focus their attention on this special approach to treatment of old patients.

In solving the problems of organisation of medical care for older age groups, the following should be borne in mind:

1. Geriatric care must be a component part of the general system of therapeutic and *prophylactic* service.
2. Geriatric care must be widely available since elderly subjects constitute a large number of the Soviet population including its working group.
3. Medical aid must be as near as possible to the elderly population by the development of dispensary-polyclinic and of home visiting services.
4. The whole system of therapeutic measures must be aimed not only to cure the pathological processes, but also to restore the general psychic state of elderly patients, to stimulate maximally and to activate mobility and ability for self-service.
5. The assessment of the organisational form and the volume of medical aid rendered to old people must be based on the population age structure, on peculiarities of its setting, its health status and other factors.

Further developments in the medical care of the elderly should look first to the complex measures required to improve the general level of therapeutic-prophylactic service, and secondly, the organisation of geriatric care. One of of the main tasks in improving the quality of medical care for old people should be the system of advanced training of physicians (primarily therapists) in gerontology and geriatrics.

In the USSR the special chair of gerontology and geriatrics was founded in the Kiev Institute for Advanced Training of Physicians in January 1970. It is concerned with improving the qualifications of physicians working in residential homes, geriatric clinics and other therapeutic and prophylactic institutions, serving mainly older individuals.

DOMICILIARY CARE

The organisation of geriatric care and special services must try to allow the older man to remain living in his own home. Life in an accustomed atmosphere amidst his belongings in steady communion with his relatives and family members keeps up his interest to the ambient world and removes the feeling of isolation.

Account must also be taken of existing trends and perspectives in housing for the elderly. The majority of old people are reluctant to become isolated in separate villages as happens in many countries. Many elderly people prefer to preserve their former residence or to move to lower storeys in the same district. To allow elderly people to go on living in their own homes various forms of extra hospital aid and of social services are to be created, including medical aid at home.

Bearing in mind a steady growth in the number of aged patients (people over 60 years old form 11.8% of the USSR population and of them 18% visit the doctor annually) and thus a large demand for medical care, one can easily understand the need to develop a trend towards geriatrics in the dispensary-polyclinic activity of medical institutions. Their structure should be modified to the growing age of their out-patients.

The demand for medical aid from the dispensary-polyclinic institutions is high among the older age groups of people (who complain of troubles of circulation, sense organs, digestion, nervous system, neoplasms, bone disease, joint and muscle disease and metabolic and allergic disturbances). The demand for medical aid in patients with circulatory diseases is 1.5 times higher than that related to any other of the above pathologies. This shows the necessity for expansion of dispensary-polyclinic aid to older patients.

In planning the volume of polyclinic aid to people aged 60 and over, one should consider from 6.9 to 7.2 visits per person per year. Because of general weakness and limited mobility an essential part of medical care should be rendered at home. For people aged 60 and over, 24-35% of visits are home visits and for those aged 80 and over 50% of all are home visits. 45% of home visits by therapeutists (doctors skilled in treatment of internal disease) are to people aged 60 and over (Chebotarev and Mankovsky 1973). Expansion of medical care at home will be achieved by increasing the number of visits by paramedical personnel. In the case of chronic diseases the physician takes indirect control over the course of treatment and of the patient's state.

Medical aid and home nursing can also provide facilities for general hygiene. These will include consultations concerning oral hygiene—fitting dentures at home—advice and help in using the toilet, in selecting clothes, footwear and in securing regular nourishment, therapeutic physical training, etc. To carry out this work among ambulant patients it is suggested that the premises of the so-called 'Rooms of Health', which have been organised in many districts in Kiev, should be used. In these premises, in order to bring medical aid near to elderly people, periodic reception hours for district therapeutists may be organised. On the same basis there may be formed a 'Group of Health' (q.v.) which both teaches hygiene and medical first aid to elderly patients and also sees that their health, household and cultural needs are met.

Alongside a wide network of medico-prophylactic institutions giving medical aid to population groups of all ages, there are in the USSR special institutions for servicing predominantly elderly persons. Geriatric institutions include geriatric consulting rooms and polyclinics which function as independent bodies or may be organised together with other therapeutic-prophylactic institutions (polyclinics, hospitals, dispensaries). In the Soviet Union about eighty geriatric consulting rooms are at work in different towns. They are centres for the organisation of medical care for elderly and old people—in effect health centres in which old people are treated for illness, with advice from various specialists—and also in which advice is given on prevention of disease. These geriatric consulting rooms are in close contact with district physicians (therapeutists), medical rooms within factories, hospitals, social welfare bodies and 'pensioners' councils. They may or may not be attached to hospitals (but most commonly they form part of the hospital out-patient clinic). Physical exercise is an important part of their activities, and in this they are associated with 'Groups of Health'. Essentially they facilitate advanced medical training in geriatrics and gerontology and maintain reguar out-patient supervision over certain population groups—old people and those of retirement age and persons with premature aging.

In many town, Kiev, Volgogard, Kislovodsk and others, geriatric consulting rooms have been organised on a social basis with active participation of physician pensioners (who have retired from full-time work). A special geriatric polyclinic is organised in Tashkent (Uzbek SSR). Apart from rendering qualified aid to geriatric patients and dispensary supervision, this polyclinic guides the activity of geriatric consulting rooms, both in Tashkent districts and in other towns of the Uzbek Republic. The activity of all geriatric institutions of the Uzbek SSR is guided by the chief geriatrist of that Republic.

The Institute of Gerontology AMS USSR has a polyclinic department. It has the following tasks:

—To afford elderly and old persons geriatric consultation. These patients are generally sent by the therapeutic and prophylactic institutions from various towns, then they are selected and hospitalised at gerontological and geriatric clinical departments for examination and treatment.

—To carry out long-term observations of certain age and occupation groups in order to discover the peculiarities of body aging at different age periods—considering also environmental factors.

—Trial and study of the efficacy of different drugs and therapeutic methods which are recommended for geriatric practice.

In the polyclinic department there is also a dispensary follow-up of those who were formerly in-patients who were included in the longitudinal studies. The polyclinic department always keeps contact with geriatric consulting rooms, pensioners and medical institutions of the town.

PREVENTIVE ASPECTS

The prophylactic work of Soviet public health and a wide development of the work of medical institutions ensures the improvement of health of the old. In prevention of premature aging (as well as improving the health of the aged), a system with widespread use of physical culture has been devised. 'Groups of Health' have found widespread expansion in the USSR and are being created at sporting organisations, therapeutic physical training dispensaries, medical institutions and at many other institutions. Physical training at these groups is proceeding according to special physiologically grounded programmes. The composition and training of each group takes into account age and state of health of the participants (the state of health being under constant medical supervision). 'Groups of Health' have nowadays become a mass physico-cultural keep-fit institution for the aged to which patients are recommended by district physicians.

Another medical development is the 'Health Zone'—this exists to maintain or restore the health of aged groups of the population and prolong their active period of life. The following are medical factors at 'Health Zones':

—Combination of a regular routine of movement, therapeutic physical training, work therapy, physical therapy and other methods.

—A mass organised holiday at city suburbs (even in the city itself). This has a health-promoting effect, particularly for the aged whose departure to remote localities is undesirable from the point of view of subsequent acclimatisation. Treatment in 'Health Zones' is performed after a complete medical examination at which, for each patient, an individual course of treatment is planned. All procedures are graded according to age and health status and carried out under supervision of a geriatric physician. At the

'Health Zone' of Baku the treatment of patients is effected without use of any drugs. The therapeutic effect is achieved by various combinations of natural cure methods, natural factors, motoregime and therapeutic physical exercises. The 'Health Zone' of Baku is organised in the area of the maritime park. It is a large medical establishment with well-equipped polyclinics including diagnostic laboratories, consulting rooms and many auxiliary medical subdivisions. Within the 'Health Zone' there are various pavilions for hydrotherapy, dietetic dining rooms, areas for supervised walking, pleasure grounds for sport, physical training, etc. The patients spend the whole day at the 'Health Zone'; the total duration of the course of treatment ranges from forty to sixty days.

'Health Zones' on a minor scale are created for single districts of towns—at parks, institutions, sporting establishments, as well as in other places where conditions are good for carrying out open air therapy and physico-culture activities. The Central 'Health Zone' is an administrative and scientific centre to guide the work of other zones. It includes a scientific centre where research into the influence of physical training, sports and other forms of treatment upon the human organism is carried out. The 'Health Zone' at Pyatigorsk was created in the local park of culture and rest. Its work is carried on under the guidance of volunteer pensioners. Medical examination of those enrolled is performed at polyclinics as is the supervision of health and of the course of treatment. Physical exercises and organisation of the motoregime are guided by a medical gymnast. Dietary nourishment is ensured by the dining room next door. Patients spend the daytime in the park pavilions equipped with chaise-longues. Definite parts of the course are devoted to favourite diversions—reading, knitting, sewing, etc.

Success of the 'Health Zone' is determined by the improvement of the general state, rise in working capacity and a decrease in morbidity. It appears to be the best way, not only of improving health, but also of providing leisure for the aged. Physical culture measures against the background of a well-established regime with work-therapy fill the pensioners' spare time with useful, meaningful occupations.

HOSPITAL CARE

The hospitalisation rate of old patients is related to the accumulation of chronic pathology with age. Only 30% of patients aged 60 and over have one disease, 40% have two diseases; the rest have three and more diseases. With increasing age, the incidence of disease detected for the first time and of acute episodes in the course of a disease is reduced. An atypical course of the disease is common and similar clinical manifestations of many diseases complicate the making of a diagnosis. A gradual change in the spectrum of prevailing diseases causes a marked 'aging' of the hospital in-patient population. Of hospitalised elderly patients 45% are for internal medicine, 11% surgical and 11% combined neurological and oncological. The urological and endocrine patients constitute a small number (5-6%). Requests for hospitalisation of people aged 60 and over is three times higher than that in the general population. (About 24-35% of people aged 60 and over each year.)

In the Soviet Union, geriatric patients are usually hospitalised in general hospitals. However, there is a number of institutions giving medical care to older patients and these are called geriatric institutions. There are 245 specialised beds at the Research Institute of Gerontology AMS, USSR for gerontology and geriatrics. These beds are used for the study of changes due to aging as well as study of the peculiarities in the development, course and treatment of diseases occurring most frequently in elderly and old persons. There is special reference to the problems of therapy and rehabilitation of such patients.

The institute includes divisions of clinical physiology and pathology, of internal organs, of the nervous system, locomotor apparatus, functional diagnosis and clinical biochemistry.

The institute clinic has also a clinical laboratory, X-ray room, physiotherapy division, hall for physical exercise, dental surgery, otolaryngologist's, urologist's rooms, etc. Apart from studying age-related peculiarities in the pathogenesis of disease the elaboration and application of the most effective therapeutic methods including new geriatric drugs is carried out.

In-patient geriatric hospital care is carried out in different types of institution. Since scanty data is available in the literature in regard to such facilities, the following figures on the trends in the development of in-patient medical care for older patients may be of particular interest. The figures (Loginova *et al.*, 1968) are as follows:

—Geriatric units within general hospitals (the need in such units is 131 per 1000 people aged 60 and over);
—Units for chronically ill patients requiring a six months' admission (81.6 per 1000 people aged 60 and over);
—Units for long-term treatment of patients suffering from irreversible forms of disease who are to stay there for a short period (29.1 per 1000 persons aged 60 and over).

Opinions vary as to the types of in-patient facility needed for long-term treatment. Further investigation into this problem is required. Since three out of four patients who need long-term care are aged 60 and over the problem of hospitals for such long-term treatment is inseparable from that of the organisation of geriatric care. Most specialists in their reports presented at many congresses and published in the journals are of the opinion that separation of old patients from younger ones requiring long-term treatment is not necessary—that organisation of units in hospitals for old people only is not jusified. This is an important organisational psychological aspect of the problem.

SOCIAL SERVICES

In creating satisfactory living conditions for aged people and improvement of their medical care, a growing role belongs to social service institutions, special homes for the aged and nursing-homes *(vide infra)*. The foundation of these institutions springs from the aging population and from altered family conditions. Every year the network of nursing-homes and the number of beds therein is growing in the USSR. Further widening of this network is foreseen by government decrees. Measures have been taken to widen this network of homes and to improve the living conditions and the medical and cultural services within them. At present the number of places in such institutions is 300 000. (Total population of Soviet Union (1970 census) is 241.7 million of which 28.5 million are aged 60 and over.) As pensions, housing and social services develop, a group of aged people who are living alone and require special services and housing becomes more apparent. This is associated with an increased demand for housing, with new measures concerned with health of the aged and with the precariousness of their nursing.

Housing for pensioners poses special problems, depending on the degree of loss of physical capacity. One group have insignificant requirements—only slight help towards their daily domestic needs. Another requires substantial aid with total exemption from household duties. A third group is not only unable to undertake domestic work, but requires domestic nursing and medical assistance.

Many old people obtaining appropriate services (supply of food products and hot meals, laundry facilities with delivery of washed linen, nursing in case of illness, etc.) can continue living in ordinary flats. For invalid patients and single persons, who due to physical or psychological conditions or for any other reasons, are unable to live either alone or with a family, special institutions (nursing-homes and boarding houses) have been created. Homes for the aged provide their inhabitants with free-of-charge board and lodging as well as with clothing, footwear, linen and medical and cultural services. These homes have their own closed system of maintenance with a definite regime.

At present there exists the following types of nursing home:

(a) Homes of ordinary type for elderly and old persons who are able to move and to satisfy, at least partly, their daily domestic needs. Such homes are provided with special premises for geriatric consulting rooms.

(b) Homes of a hospital type for sick persons who have chronic illness, mostly bed-ridden and who require constant nursing and medical aid

(c) Homes for psycho-geriatric or mentally disordered patients who are to be isolated from healthy people.

In recent years with increased pensions as well as improved housing, homes for the aged are settled mostly by sick persons who require constant nursing and medical help. The group of practically healthy persons in them does not exceed 16%. More than 84% of those in homes are in need of systematic medical supervision, treatment and nursing. 45% of them require constant in-patient treatment, special medical care and rehabilitation therapy. As far as pathology is concerned, patients in nursing-homes resemble those who require long-term treatment and hospitalisation.

The inhabitants of homes for the aged obtain both in-patient and out-patient medical aid. Systematic examination of residents' state of health is practised as well as dispensary supervision over the groups requiring therapy. Measures for general hygiene and prevention of infection are taken. In a typical home for bed-ridden patients, special wards similar to those for chronic patients at hospitals are foreseen.

Homes for the aged are also provided with an X-ray room, physiotherapy, dental surgery and clinical laboratories in proportion to their size. In many homes for the aged work therapy is used as a therapeutic factor. Residents who have relatively good health are allowed to work in sewing workshops, in the gardens, in flower growing shops, weaving shops, etc.

The capacity of homes for the aged varies but most are for 100, 150 or 500 residents. Both small and large homes have their merits and de-merits. The small home has psychological advantages; it can be furnished to look like an ordinary flat. A large home has more facilities for organising cultural and medical services and is more economic. For various towns different sizes of homes are recommended. For middle and large-sized towns, homes with a capacity of 150-200 places: for great cities - of 300-400 places and more. It is practicable to settle the homes with people from the local population. Sites for building homes are usually allotted close to park areas with satisfactory communication to housing districts of the town.

Types of care for the elderly in USSR

Preventive care
- 'Group of Health' (in rooms of health and in geriatric consulting rooms)
- 'Health Zone'
- University of Health and Longevity in Kiev

Domiciliary care
- Polyclinic
- Rooms of health (in Kiev only)
- Geriatric consulting rooms

Hospital care
- Geriatric units in general hospitals
- Medium-term chronically ill
- Long-term treatment

Nursing-homes
- Residential
- Chronically disabled
- Psycho-geriatrics

HEALTH EDUCATION

At present when in many countries the number of old people is increasing, many prefer to live in their own homes. Being ill themselves or taking care of sick relatives, they need knowledge of health matters and some medical education. There is no doubt that along with a rise of general hygiene it is necessary to educate people in skills of self-service and service to others, as well as some knowledge of care of the sick. It is important that the old should be taught how to plan the daily routine with a correct alternation of work and leisure; motor activity and balanced nutrition accorded to age and health. The final goal of all this activity should be a prolongation of active, meaningful life span, preservation of mobility, ability for self-service and maintenance of a good psycho-physical state.

Among the varying forms of health education of the old age groups is the University of Health and Longevity in Kiev. Studies are for five to six persons at a time, held in the polyclinic departments and in-patient units of the Institute of Gerontology AMS, USSR. The Institute has ten years' experience of holding courses with older population groups at the City Public University, Health and Longevity. The aim of this University is to convey systematic knowledge on the most important hygienic and medical questions to those taking part by a course of monthly lectures.

The material presented should incorporate the latest ideas in gerontology and geriatrics, including on the one hand information about a healthy environment in which older people may live and on the other, recommendations about the health promoting activities. Some lectures are followed by practical lessons, e.g. demonstration of exercises, exhibition and advice on cooking, food, use of herbs, etc. Periodically consultations are held with geriatrists of different specialties (eye specialists, neurologists, dieticians, etc.). Such studies finish with an entertainment programme (concert or film demonstration). At the closing session questions are asked and answered followed by a ceremonial granting of a diploma. Organisation of Universities of Health and Longevity can be recommended as one of the effective means of advanced medical training for elderly people.

References

Chebotarev, F. and Mankovsky, N. B. (eds.) (1973). *Geriatrics*

Loginova, E. A., Potekhira, M. V. *et al.* (1968). *Problems of Medico-Social Aid to the Elderly,* 48-52 Institute for Social Hygiene and Organisation of Public Health named after N. A. Semashko (Meditsina, Moscow: Sovetskoye Zdravookhranenije, No. 10)

CHAPTER SEVEN

Australia

R M Gibson

HISTORY

Medical care for old people in Australia began in the obscurity of the original colonial society. Early European settlers in Australia were transported from England and penal colonies were established. The European background of local government was non-existent and no equivalent of the English Poor Laws of the 1830s was established. The care of the aged rested with each individual family, but for the 'beginning' assistance, provided by the early charity organistions which began to function in several of the colonies in the 1830s. Some of these charities were subsidised in part by colonial governments. The recipients of charitable aid were those judged as 'worthy' people and a punitive attitude was evident towards the elderly who were disabled and poor.

In general, the early Australian society had no affluent leisure class who could provide money to endow the carc of the aged or find the time to be involved in voluntary work. In this early environment the various colonial governments began to make their own provisions for social services generally and the economic depression of the 1890s stimulated political awareness of the need for government involvement.

In 1901, both the state of Victoria and New South Wales introduced an old age pension and the state of Queensland followed in 1908. In the same year, The Commonwealth Government introduced old age pensions subject to means test. These were the days of Federation and the Constitution written for the Federation of the Sovereign States of Australia (Commonwealth of Australia) whilst centralising many powers in the

Federal Government left residual unspecified powers to the states. For example, education, health, housing and care of the destitute remained state matters and remained centralised at state level with little or no involvement of local government. The Commonwealth aged pension continues to be paid subject to means test. However, at the time of writing, the means test is being progressively tapered with the eventual object of abolition. It has been stated by Federal Governments, and this by both Government and opposition parties, that policy is to progressively abolish all means tests for aged pensions.

The level of monetary payments vary upwards from time to time with a loose relationship to the minimum legal wage. The object is to provide an 'adequate subsistance allowance' assuming that the pensioner has the usual capital resources of home, car and a specified maximum in cash savings. Where home rental is paid by the pensioner, a rental subsidy is added to the pension and where the recipient is over 80 years of age, an additional 'personal care' allowance is added.

For these reasons then the medical care of old people developed along many different lines in the various states. Some developed State Hospitals administered by the State Public Health Department, others encouraged Benevolent, Church and other charitable organisations to do this work.

FACILITIES AND FINANCE

In Queensland and Tasmania particularly and to some extent in New South Wales, state hospitals for the aged were established whereas in Victoria particularly large Benevolent Institutions developed both in the capital city of Melbourne and in rural Victoria.

Since 1910, there have been periodic considerations of contributing schemes and a Royal Commission investigated the proposition of national insurance covering, among other matters, old age and invalidity. However, no action has ever been taken on this question and, in fact, in this year of 1974 the question is still being debated at Federal level.

The day-to-day medical care of the elderly rested virtually in the hands of the private medical practitioner who gave of his time and skill in an honorary capacity both in the community and in the hospitals and other institutions.

Up to and following the 1914-1918 war, there had been a steady growth of privately owned nursing-homes run for profit where the more affluent elderly could receive basic medical and nursing care. In New South Wales—in the relative absence of extensive government hospitals or benevolent institutions—private nursing-homes flourished and continue to do so. The result is that now over 50% of private nursing-homes for the aged in Australia are situated in the state of New South Wales. In 1973 Australia had 50.2 nursing-home beds per 1000 population of 65 years and over 17.8 aged person hostel beds per 1000 aged population. (A total of 68 beds per 1000 population aged 65 and over.) It has been recommended that the combined figure should be reduced to 40 per 000 made up of 20 per 000 nursing-home and 20 per 000 hostel beds. The reason behind this is that where the alternative of hostel accommodation is not available then 'hostel type' patients enter nursing-homes. Thus some people in nursing-homes could and should live in hostels if these were available as an alternative.

The population of Australia at the last census (1973) was 13 million of whom 8.4% were aged 65 and over. Immigration following the 1914-1918 war increased Australia's population by some 3 million people over thirty years. Many of these were assisted immigrants from Britain who brought with them the concept of prepaid medical care in the form of 'Friendly Societies' and the 'Doctor Club'. These were private contractual arrangements between an individual—a family or a friendly society—and a doctor to provide a stated range of medical care in return for an agreed total fee for an agreed period of time. In many cases medicines were dispensed within the same arrangement.

Following the 1939-1945 war a system of Federal Government subsidised voluntary contributing health insurance was introduced in Australia and 'Fee for Service' medical practice became common. Here the doctors' fee was paid partly by Commonwealth Government subsidy and partly by the relevant health insurance company. The patient was responsible for any amount in excess of this combined rebate. At the same time the Commonwealth Government introdued the 'Pensioners Medical Service' on a national basis. A doctor could apply to be recognised by the government for this purpose and agreed to provide day-to-day care for the pensioner for a standard fee for each service, paid by the Federal Government. The pensioner must present himself at a public hospital for specialist services when these are needed. These specialised services were provided at public hospitals largely by visiting honorary specialists supported on some occasions by junior house staff (resident medical officer). It is only in recent years that Public General Hospitals have begun to build up a proportion of full-time paid specialist staff. Under these conditions the medical care for old people has been largely in the hands of family doctors with access to specialist consultation which was limited, especially if the patient was not ambulant (e.g. in a nursing-home). Thus no career prospect exists to encourage physicians to qualify themselves as specialists in geriatric medicine since a specialist could not belong to the 'Pensioners Medical Service'.

At present only limited prospects in salaried positions exist to encourage the development of the speciality of geriatric medicine. Differing financial arrangements for the medical care of old people limits freedom of movement between such medical care resources as acute general hospital beds, nursing-home, long-stay geriatric hospitals and hostels for the aged. Many are accommodated in general hospital beds who could more properly be treated in nursing-homes or long-stay geriatric hospitals: many occupy nursing-home beds who could manage in sheltered hostels or community supported home care programmes.

Financial arrangements differ from resource to resource and are different in different states except that the medical and hospital care of the age-pensioner in Australia generally is free to him. His pension continues to be paid and he may dispose of it as he wishes. All hospital care to everybody is free in the state of Queensland and the Federal Government is at present considering free 'Standard Ward Accommodation' in all public general hospitals in Australia. This would be financed from general tax (Federal income tax) revenue and dispensed to the hospitals on a bed/day occupancy basis. Both the hospitals (except state hospitals) and the states are uncertain of the future of this kind of arrangement since subsidy from government sources often lags behind current costs—especially in an inflationary financial climate.

The elderly citizen who, by reason of his means, does not qualify for the old-age pension, is encouraged to cover the costs of possible hospitalisation in a general hospital or a licenced private hospital by voluntary contribution to a registered hospital insurance organisation. Rebate from this should he be hospitalised, covers the greater proportion of hospital accommodation cost. He should also cover himself separately against any charges made by his attending doctor. In state owned geriatric long-stay hospitals and in some non-profit benevolent long-stay facilities the age-pensioner is charged a proportion of his pension and retains some as 'pocket money'. The proportions vary (e.g. 60% of pension taken as fees, 40% retained by pensioner). This proportion of his pension does not cover the cost of the bed; the remainder is paid for by the state.

Of recent times in the state of New South Wales it was estimated that non-profit Benevolent Home care cost the charitable society 60 cents per day over and above the total of pension and bed/day subsidy paid by the Federal Government. To offset this trend the Federal subsidy has been increased. In the private nursing-home sector the effect of fixing fees and subsidy has led to a near crisis situation. Wages of staff and other costs have risen so that nursing-homes are threatening closure. The pensioner in the private nursing-home must be supported financially by his family to meet the costs of his care.

STAFF

The basic unit of treatment and care in all forms of hospital bed is the nurse and increasingly in Australia do we see the employment of the 'Nurse Aide' or 'Assistant in Nursing' as a patient-care labour force. Training programmes leading to a certificate of registration within a particular state are increasingly offered to the nursing-aide. Student nurses proceeding to Registered Nurse Certificate are also employed in general hospitals and a special course, either primary or 'bridging' from another nursing discipline, in geriatric nursing is offered in several states (e.g. New South Wales).

In general terms there is an overall shortage of paramedical staff—social workers, physiotherapists, occupational therapists and speech therapists. In some situations these paramedical disciplines have agreed to the supervised employment of 'aide' staff, but except in social work, no formal training has yet been offered to these 'aides'. In Sydney and in Newcastle, New South Wales, colleges of technical education have begun training courses for 'Social Welfare Officers' who, it is hoped will support the professionally trained paramedical specialists. Such professional paramedical personnel as exist tend to concentrate in capital cities leaving provincial centres and rural towns without their services.

For the above reasons hospital care and in the near future also community care for the elderly rests heavily on the nurse and her 'aide' staff. Therefore, the most urgent priority for the future of geriatric treatment in Australia revolves around the education of the nurse in modern geriatric treatment methods.

University teaching hospitals and general hospitals in Australia have not recognised a role for themselves in modern geriatrics. This, in the opinion of the writer, is because of the lack of career prospects for a specialist geriatrician who should stimulate and lead such activity, both in teaching and in developing services. There have been a few notable exceptions to this rule in that some large general hospitals in Australia have applied themselves to the development of departments of geriatric medicine and they have conducted hospital and community programmes in geriatrics. In all such cases the departments have been developed and administered by full-time salaried physicians specialising in geriatrics. Mention must be made of some of these because their activities are likely to provide the basic models in any future development. For example, the

Royal Newcastle Hospital, Newcastle, New South Wales, began its service with acute general ward care, geriatric rehabilitation and assessment followed by (and controlling) a comprehensive community-supporting service in Newcastle in 1955. Other notable developments include the Princess Alexandra Hospital in Brisbane, Queensland; the Sir Charles Gardnair Hospital in Perth, Western Australia; and the Lidcombe Hospital in Sydney, New South Wales. At the time of writing, there is only one University teaching post in geriatric medicine in Australia and that is held by Professor R. B. LeFroy in Perth, Western Australia.

There has been little significant involvement of the medical undergraduate or the hospital intern in geriatric medicine. In general terms the acute general hospital bed is cleared of geriatric patients by exporting them to nursing-homes, or, with little rehabilitation or assessment, to community care resources which may be ill equipped to manage the problems presented to them.

CONCEPTS OF CARE

In the geriatric units in hospitals offering acute restorative treatment two definitely differing philosophies may be discovered. One is the 'gymnasium' oriented programmes involving paramedical staff on a person-to-person treatment basis with very little, if any, involvement of the nurse. These are similar in many respects to the general rehabilitation units common in most advanced countries but have been adapted to the treatment of the elderly. In these programmes it is felt that the daily life of the patient is 'disability orientated' and may lead to frustration when full functional recovery is not achieved. The patient may have difficulty in translating exercise into function and the nurse, to whose care he returns at the end of his treatment session, having not been involved, is unaware of the necessary techniques and attitudes to continue his treatment for the rest of the day or the week. Nursing morale is likely to suffer and the nurse to remain 'sickness orientated'.

The other is the 'function orientated' programme in which the patient's geriatric retraining is built into his daily living. In this type of programme nurses, at all levels, are fully involved. They are supervised, guided and educated by a nurse trained in geriatric nursing, supported very closely by the paramedical specialists. In this programme the patient's abilities are emphasised, function is recovered within the limit of residual disability and the nurse sees the product of her work.

It is noted that the 'gymnasium orientated' programme is most seen where the supply of paramedical staff is good and the 'function orientated' programme where paramedical personnel are scarce.

It is felt that in Australia, generally, with its rural communities and predictable continuing scarcity of paramedical personnel, the 'function orientated' type of programme should be encouraged.

It must be appreciated that the aims and, therefore, the reason for existence of special geriatric units is to prepare patients, usually, for return to community living. For this reason their retraining activities must be 'reality orientated' and closely coordinated with community supportive services. A model along these lines has existed in Newcastle, New South Wales since 1955. This model is based on and controlled by the Royal Newcastle Hospital and the hospital and community service is directed by a specialist in geriatric medicine supported by a multi-disciplinal staff of paramedical and nursing colleagues. The basic concepts of this model have been applied in a few other centres in Australia, e.g. Princess Alexandra Hospital in Brisbane, Queensland; the Lidcombe Hospital in Sydney, New South Wales; and the Sir Charles Gardnair Hospital in Perth, Western Australia.

In other situations, community supportive care of the disabled elderly has been supplied by visiting nursing services unrelated to hospital care. The oldest of these are traditionally community based services such as the Royal Sydney District Nursing Service, the Royal Melbourne District Nursing Service, the Silver Chain organisation in West Australia and the 'Blue Nurses' organisation in Queensland. In South Australia, community supportive services grew out of the activities of a delivered meals service services grew out of the activities of a delivered meals service (Meals-on-Wheels Incorporated of South Australia). Elsewhere local government bodies have subsidised or directly employed visiting nurses who, whilst having a generalist function, are mainly occupied with the domestic nursing support of the disabled elderly. In general these services are supported financially by charitable donations helped in some instances by local government, State government and Commonwealth government subsidy. In one instance the community nursing service has been accepted for funding purposes as a general hospital and receives funds from its state health commission as if it were a general hospital. That is, its income is derived from such sources as fees, charitable donations and money grant from state government. It is the opinion of the writer that many of these community-based visiting nurse services are professionally unsupported and do not relate to the range of resources necessary for them to perform their desired role. In too many instances do their supportive services serve only to maintain an unsatisfactory 'care' role with little exposure to remedial treatment.

In remote rural situations supportive care for the disabled elderly is provided at a small cottage hospital staffed in some instances by a 'Bush

Nursing' organisation in turn supported by the Royal Flying Doctor Service which operates using a widespread radio communication service and aerial transport. The medical care of the elderly Australian Aboriginal is an unsolved problem in remote areas and involves such factors as detribalisation, lack of acceptance and still a somewhat nomadic life. The incidence of visual defect is said to be high in the nomadic elderly aboriginal. Contributing factors are the corneal lesions (opacity of the lower half of the cornea due to exposure to ultraviolet light in plains and desert people), trachoma and of recent times the visual stigmata of diabetes mellitus.

In some cities (and in fact only in some parts of some cities) other community supportive services are available, e.g. delivered meals, home-helps and socially supportive club activity. In provincial centres and country towns there has been in recent years, an awakening community awareness of the community responsibility to its aged citizens so that one sees the beginning development of common supportive services. Charity organisations, local government and recently Federal government are becoming increasingly involved.

Such organisations as the Australian Association of Gerontology and more recently the Australian Geriatrics Society have been concerned with both education and some research into the welfare of the aged and the Australian Council on Aging has played an increasing role in the encouragement of overall welfare needs. Forward developments in the care of old people in Australia at this time are in a most fluid state and depend to a large extent on current political conflict in the National Parliament. The question of contributory National Health Insurance is again raised, the proposed activities of the National Health and Hospitals Commission and the National Social Welfare Commissions are awaiting political decisions in relation to funds. If funded, these commissions propose to finance local community health and welfare activity. In some cases direct grants may be made, in others funds may be paid through State Health Authorities for special purposes.

Activities concerned with medical and social welfare of the elderly include housing, frail aged hostels, community day care centres, community nursing, etc. Several states have Directors of Geriatrics in their health departments. Others have senior advisors in geriatrics. The state of New South Wales has recently declared identifiable health regions with a large degree of decentralised authority vested in a Regional Director of Health. Some of these Regional Directors have Regional Geriatricians as senior advisors on their staff. In some regions the Regional Geriatrician has a number of community physicians in geriatrics. Each community physician heads a multidisciplinary team of nurses, social workers, occupational therapists, physiotherapists and speech therapists. He has access to treatment beds both in acute general hospital and in rehabilitation and can mobilise such supportive community services as delivered meals, home-help and day care, etc. He works as a consultant to general practitioners and to other medical agencies, e.g. hospitals and nursing-homes. This recent development is an example of repeating the Newcastle model adapted to local community needs.

It is hoped that a proliferation of this concept will enable local need to be met and effective liaison and coordination between the various care-giving agencies to be established and maintained.

Reference

Sax, S. (1969). *Medical Care in the Melting Pot* (London, Australia: Angus and Robertson).

CHAPTER EIGHT

Conclusion

J C Brocklehurst

There can be no doubt about the size of the commitment which looms before all advanced societies in providing medical care for old people both now and throughout the rest of this century. Individual statistics in all the chapters provide sufficient evidence of this. The need, therefore, is to try and discern which among the various approaches seems to offer the best results, both in terms of value for money and also in the humanity of the care provided.

Except for the USSR all the other chapters have described the development of care on the basis of a capitalist society and it is clear that this may happen in one of two ways—either by gradual evolution, as is most apparent in the United States of America and in Australia; or by revolution, i.e. the setting up of a state service, as is evident in Great Britain and to a lesser extent in Sweden. The position of the Netherlands would seem to lie midway between these two opposites. The development of medical care for old people by gradual evolution means that it will be considerably influenced by the political power of the providers, especially the medical associations and the owners of nursing-homes and hospitals. These will pull in one direction and it is likely that the state whose immediate function will be to supply finance, but who by doing this cannot but influence developmental policy, will pull in the other and the product available to the patient will be the equilibrium between these two forces. The problem of different types of financial arrangements preventing the optimal movement of elderly patients through different types of care has been well brought out and as Rossman indicates, for instance, the nature of a professional service such as domiciliary nursing available to a patient may depend on whether or not the particular *procedure* qualifies for payment.

These matters, of course, affect, although to a lesser extent, the provision of care in those countries where a comprehensive service has come about by 'revolution'. Here on the whole the patient may be able to progress more smoothly from one stage of care to the next, but even here the source of finance may cause problems, as in the long waiting time (in Great Britain) engendered between patients moving from hospital geriatric departments (financed by the National Health Service) to old people's residential homes (financed by the local authority).

It must be remembered that nowadays only a very rich old person could provide independently and privately for all his needs when he is ill, particularly when that illness leads to long-term disability and that, disease in old age tends to be long-term and disabling rather than acute and fully recoverable. Therefore, progressive care through departments (or facilities) providing acute, intermediate (rehabilitation) and then either long-stay or domiciliary care is likely to be needed most commonly.

To achieve a smooth passage through these various stages implies a unified or coordinated administration and is perhaps one of the best arguments for a specialist service of geriatric medicine which can assume responsibility for the ill old person at an early stage and steer him through all the subsequent stages until his resettlement in the community, or in the most appropriate type of long-term care. By this means a uniformity of approach and a continued flow of information about the patient should have the best chance of happening.

It is clear that in all the nations under consideration the emergence of a specialty of geriatric medicine has been slow and in most of them has met with considerable antagonism from the medical establishment. The USSR Great Britain and Sweden all now have established specialists in significant numbers but in the other countries there are only very few and these largely individuals who have become specialists on a personal basis because they have found themselves, in whatever appointments they may hold, to have been mainly dealing with old people. That antagonism towards the specialty still exists even in Great Britain, where it is now firmly grounded with 300 state-employed specialists and eight university chairs, is evidenced from the difficulties in obtaining staff (particularly potential trainees): this in itself is likely to be a reflection of the attitudes of older and more senior doctors.

In Great Britain and the United States the paradox exists of a gross shortage of medical practitioners supplemented by large numbers of immigrant doctors in a situation where many young people leaving school are qualified to study medicine and would wish to do so, yet are unable to find places in medical schools. This shortage of personnel inevitably reflects most heavily on specialties like geriatric medicine which are therefore, unable to reach their full potential.

It is not easy to account for the antagonism towards geriatrics except on the basis of a value judgement concerning the medical needs of people towards the end of their lives. Yet it is clear that because of multiple and long-term disabilities this is one of the most medically complex stages of life and one in which the trained specialist can develop a whole spectrum of care, including day hospital, rehabilitative and long-term care in addition to acute and episodic care, in a way that no generalist is able or indeed prepared to consider doing.

Of course, there is a vicious circle in the fact that old age, being the least valued part of life, attracts poor resources and such inadequate facilities make the whole field of care seem less attractive to doctors.

The overwhelming arguments in favour of a specialist service would seem to be (*a*) the size of the problem (*b*) the neglect it suffers when there is no such service (*c*) the many clinical and organisational improvements that have occurred where a service has been established and (*d*) the fact that those who engage in it find the work exciting, stimulating and worthwhile.

PRIMARY CARE

One striking difference between the various countries described lies in the attitudes towards medical visiting of old people at home. It seems that in the United States it is almost impossible to have an old person visited at home by a doctor, except in the pioneering schemes such as those described by Rossman at Montefiore. In Sweden also home consultations have almost disappeared. In Great Britain and the USSR on the other hand, medical consultations in old people's homes still form a very important part of the system of medical care for old people. A high proportion of patients admitted to geriatric departments in Britain are seen first by the specialist geriatrician as well as by the general practitioner at home and in many cases alternative arrangements may be made instead of admission—such as the use of a day hospital, out-patient attendance, etc. There is thus a balance between these two trends but because of the frailty and disability of so many ill old people and because of the important part which their home environment plays in their future progress, it would seem that the case for home consultation is a strong one.

EDUCATION

The training of doctors in handling the problems of old people mirrors the degree of commitment to a geriatric service, thus in both Great Britain and Sweden, professional training for these specialists is clearly laid down and the length and manner of training is the same as for other medical specialties. The teaching to undergraduates of the principles of geriatric medical practice is also gradually evolving and at the present time is most developed in the USSR and Great Britain. It seems that the medical curriculum evolves with enormous slowness and there may be some merit in this. However, it is hard to see why it should not lay its greatest emphasis on the areas of medical practice which are going to involve the greatest amount of doctors' time once they are qualified; there can be no doubt that one of these areas is medicine in old age.

The education of old people themselves has been especially emphasised by Revutskaya. Whether the maintenance of health in old age by physical exercise and gymnastics, periodic visits to a Health Zone (that is, in effect, a recuperative and reinvigorating holiday) and the provision of attractive pastimes should be the province of the Health or Education Services is perhaps a matter for debate. What cannot be doubted is that there is every reason to encourage old people to engage in these activities and every expectation that by so doing they cannot but gain in mental and physical health.

A further aspect of training is the gradual emergence of aides, more particularly for nurses but also, as indicated by Rossman, as physician substitutes. This is happening to some extent in all the countries described and various categories of special workers are emerging; for instance, in Holland there are nursing-aides for the elderly with a two year training and similarly in Australia.

Finally, one of the greatest problem areas within the field of geriatric medicine itself is the care of the mentally deteriorated old person and in particular the sufferer from senile dementia. In Great Britain large numbers of these patients are maintained at home, often at the expense of considerable strain on relatives and families. In Holland it is suggested that there should be homes for them combined with those for physically frail old people. In the United States and Great Britain there is a declared policy of closing the large mental hospitals built in the 19th Century, usually beyond the city limits. It is, however, quite unrealistic to attempt to do this in the face of increasing mental morbidity among the elderly, without providing clear alternatives. The use of the day hospital may help in the control of this problem and the development of psychiatrists with their special or total interest in psychiatry of old age cannot but be welcome.

Perhaps in relation to the single symptom of mental confusion the need for accurate and comprehensive diagnosis is most obviously demonstrated. This applies to all illness and disability in old age and is the reason why, whatever course of care is planned for an old person in our advanced society, it must be based on the most careful medical assessment, followed by the easy and rapid availability of the type of care most suitable for each individual's unique problems.

Index